THE
TRAIL
RUNNING
GUIDEBOOK

*For all trail runners
who want to **Perform Wilder***

HANNY ALLSTON

Second Female, Ultra-Trail Australia 100 km 2017
Winner, Ultra-Trail Australia 50 km 2016
Record Holder, Six Foot Track Marathon 2015
Record Holder, Overland Track Ultra 2013

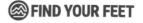

Find Your Feet
107 Elizabeth Street, Hobart, Tasmania, 7000
Australia

findyourfeet.com.au

Published October 2018.

ISBN
Paperback: 978-0-6483929-0-3
Mobi: 978-0-6483929-1-0
Epub: 978-0-6483929-2-7

Managing editor: Belinda Pollard
Proofreader: Alix Kwan

CAUTION

I am not a doctor but rather a coach drawing from
professional and personal experiences. I am writing
this book for you based on this understanding. It will
require you to listen to your body as well as the advice of other professionals around you. Furthermore,
you should always consult your doctor or allied
health professional before beginning a new exercise
program.

Reactions to *The Trail Running Guidebook*

Darryl Griffiths, author & founder, Shotz Sports Nutrition Australia: For every action there is a positive and/or negative reaction. This certainly rings true with Hanny's philosophy of life and running. Hanny covers all areas of mind and body, with a sound understanding that we are all unique and there is no 'one size fits all'. This book is the go-to for any level of runner from beginner to elite.

> 'This book is the go-to for any level of runner from beginner to elite.'
> Darryl Griffiths

Hannah Clark, elite Australian lightweight rower turned distance runner: I came to Hanny years ago with a simple request – to help me to train for a trail marathon in the Swiss Alps. I had no idea that out of this would come not just a fantastic athletic experience, but the beginning of a relationship that would truly change my life. At the time, on paper I was a successful athlete, having represented my country on the international stage. The reality, however, was an individual who was over-worked, over-stressed, and broken. Years of following punishing, prescriptive training plans meant that I had lost my athletic intuition, my joy in movement, and even my sense of self.

Hanny's training philosophy is worlds away from the accepted performance paradigm. Punishment is not the only way to achieve success. In fact, Hanny's methods will enable you to see that through finding your sense of play and wonder, you can achieve greater things than you ever thought possible. This is the training philosophy for the real person – where the stress of work, family and general life is actually accounted for. Whatever your version of 'success' is – whether that be elite performance or simply to get moving in the mountains – Hanny will help you to achieve just that.

> 'Punishment is not the only way to achieve success. Hanny's methods will enable you to see that through finding your sense of play and wonder, you can achieve greater things.'
> Hannah Clark

I hope you will find, as I did, that the positive impact of playing, performing and being 'wilder' will extend far beyond just athletic performance. Hanny has truly helped me to find my feet – in sport, and in life. So set your sights on your next adventure, feel your toes start to tingle with excitement and anticipation, and head off in the direction of your goal. I think that out there on the trails you'll find your feet – and even more.

Kellie Gibson, mother & businesswoman: I chose Hanny's training planner in the lead up to the 2018 Ultra-Trail Australia 22 km. For me, it was the obvious choice in my return to longer racing after a period of burnout and recurring injuries. This was due to a combination of overtraining and life stressors.

Initially I had chosen the program to allow me to get through the training and event in one piece, but was blown away by the performance gains I made along the way. This meant shifting the goal posts and my expectations on what I could achieve on race day.

I thoroughly enjoyed following the Wave Training and always looked forward to the next session. The well-balanced approach of the structure allowed me to gain confidence throughout my training while providing adequate recovery and adaptation time between key sessions. This ensured I hit the start line feeling prepared, fresh, fit and confident, which is something I had failed to achieve for a very long time!

Hanny's training program and this guidebook really exceeded my expectations. The guidebook was an excellent go-to for problem solving my challenges as they came up in training, such as nutrition and fuelling. I would recommend this program and guidebook to anyone preparing for a trail event who is wanting a well-balanced approach that is achievable in terms of volume while still making performance gains. Hanny's program offers something for everyone and can be easily adapted to runners of all levels, lifestyles and goals. My confidence and motivation has continued to soar post the 22 km event! This is the best investment I have made in my running in a very long time.

> 'I had chosen the program to allow me to get through the training and event in one piece, but was blown away by the performance gains I made along the way.' Kellie Gibson

Bonnie Davies, athlete & shift-working nurse: Recently I competed in my first trail marathon in South Africa.

Apart from the occasional fun trot on the trails or short cross-country events, I really am largely committed to road running. Prior to the event I sought the advice and assistance of Hanny. Hanny provided valuable advice and also a copy of *The Trail Running Guidebook.* This book was my bible! I read and absorbed it, making notes. I took it with me, cramming the night before the event. I ran the event with Hanny's words fresh in my mind and they were worth their weight in gold – or silver, as I came in second female and sixth overall! Thank you Hanny.

> 'Hanny's words ... were worth their weight in gold – or silver, as I came in second female and sixth overall!'
> Bonnie Davies

Erika Brann, athlete & working mother: Some people have the ability to make you believe you can conquer the world. Hanny is one of those people. Whether it is a short conversation, a mentoring session, or even reading her blog, you come away thinking, 'Yes, I can! When can I start?' Not only has Hanny helped me to achieve my running goals, more importantly she has given me the confidence to believe and trust in my own ability. She has empowered me to make smarter training decisions for myself and to realise that I am in the driver's seat. I have found the Wave Training Theory

> 'Some people have the ability to make you believe you can conquer the world. Hanny is one of those people.'
> Erika Brann

easy to follow and manipulate into my busy life. And I long for those Mission weeks! Her nutrition advice has helped me summit volcanoes, mountains and many ultra-running events. I really have come to realise that running well is so much more than just a spreadsheet. I believe that with the help of all Hanny's resources, including the podcasts tours and this guidebook, she has helped me to nurture my true self.

Dr Chris Hayes, Pain Medicine Specialist: Hanny Allston has a passion for the planet's wilder places and helping people to access them in relative safety. She has the gift of making her experience as an elite athlete understandable to the recreational trail runner. Endurance trail running will always involve discomfort, but applying the distilled wisdom of this guidebook will undoubtedly minimise the pain.

> 'She has the gift of making her experience as an elite athlete understandable to the recreational trail runner.'
> Dr Chris Hayes

In loving memory of Max and Jackie,
who inspired me to learn and love
the art of running.

Foreword

HANNY ALLSTON HAS BEEN MY MENTOR, FRIEND AND go-to girl for all things running since I attended one of her running camps in February 2015. Through her positive guidance, in a few years I have gone from being a novice runner thrilled to finish a 50 km, to competing in an international 175 km mountain race, the 2017 Ultra-Trail du Mont-Blanc, where I finished 23rd female.

Following Hanny's training principles for every race has allowed me to stand on start lines feeling confident that I have covered all the bases. More importantly, it has let me manage injuries so I can race to my full potential.

Hanny's Wave Training Theory allows the body time to recover from hard sessions, limiting the risk of injury. It also promotes a natural ebb and flow of intensity so that I'm mentally eager on the hard weeks, knowing recovery is just around the corner. But by far the best thing about the training structure is Mission Day! These are the times I go to the mountains with friends and remember that trail running is SO MUCH FUN!

When it comes to racing, I've faced sizeable nutrition & hydration challenges. If you are someone who has stood on the side of the trail puking, you will appreciate how vital these sections of *The Trail Running Guidebook* are going to be!

Hanny's 'big picture' approach makes her a great educator. From her own athletic experience and professional background, she understands the importance of weaving together physical training, recovery, mental state, nutrition & hydration, gear requirements and injury management.

Wherever you are in your running journey, let this guidebook inspire you to grab your shoes and go!

Brook Martin
From recreational athlete to elite international trail runner
23rd Female, Ultra-Trail du Mont-Blanc 100 mile 2017
6th Female, Ultra-Trail Cape Town 100 km 2017
6th Female, Ultra-Trail Australia 100 km 2018

Acknowledgements

THIS BOOK IS AN ACCUMULATION OF THE KNOWLedge, skills and beliefs that I have developed throughout my elite racing and coaching careers. I use the word 'accumulation' because these lessons have come from trial and error, asking questions and seeking answers, and also the wisdom and support of a number of people whom I am fortunate to call my mentors, friends and family.

To my earliest coaches who instilled in me a willingness to try, thank you.

To Max, who willed me to work hard, run lightly, dream boldly and consistently reminded me that there is no such word as 'cannot'. Your teachings will always influence me.

To Jackie, who listened when I needed an ear, imparted lessons from her personal experiences, and saw me as both Hanny and as an athlete. I miss you.

To my family, friends and support networks who have shared this journey, believing in me even in my own moments of doubt. You have all had a big influence on my ability to Be, Play and Perform Wilder.

To my book coach and editor, Belinda. You have given my words a presence and a space to celebrate. Thank you for sharing your knowledge and skills.

To my husband, Graham... my best friend and business partner, too. You truly have helped me to find both my feet and my voice. Furthermore, you have helped me reconnect with my love of wilder adventures, a space which never ceases to teach me some of the hardest and yet most beautiful lessons. May our wilder missions continue till we are greyer, older, and wobbling along uneven trails.

Hanny Allston

Contents

- - - - - - - - - - -

1. Perform Wilder

I<small>N MY MOST ELITE RACING YEARS, SUCCESS WAS ABOUT</small> times, results, performances. Not any more! Today my very personal definition of success is: **a willingness to reach the edge of discomfort and be willing to play there.**

What is your definition?

The Find Your Feet *Trail Running Guidebook* is a summary of my personal coaching methodologies with a focus on sustainable, long-term health and training successes. My focus is on helping you to 'find your feet'. I am interested in *you*. Embarking on wild adventures or entering races is about starting on a journey that will require patience and, hopefully, a very, very long-term approach.

I hope that the success of your own performances and aspiration is measured by: the health and adventures you have along the way; the spontaneity you create within the training structures you apply; and the *'What next?'* you ask yourself in the weeks after your chosen goal. Notice how my measure of success is not the finishing time or crossing of the finish line of a race?

I have learnt through hard lessons that racing success does not make you a better or more successful person. Rather, the journey and the 'self' you build along the way are better measures of personal attainment. Make whatever goal you set yourself a transition into a life of playful adventure, done in a way that will be sustainable until a day that is a long, long way into the future!

Be Wilder, Play Wilder and Perform Wilder

My coaching and personal philosophy has arisen from years of coaching a wide array of recreational athletes, as well as my own experiences performing among elite athletes across a breadth of sports, from swimming to orienteering, marathon running to ultra-distance trail racing.

I believe that performance occurs when there is a union of an individual's sense of self, their ability to find joy in the pursuit, and the consistency of their preparation, knowledge, and experiences. It is a pinnacle, the tip of your athletic pathway at a given moment in time. It requires you to be ready to be there: mentally, physically, but also emotionally. For you to reach this pinnacle in the first place, you must have done the work and then have been willing to put it all out on the line on the day. This requires an absolute love of what you do, but also an incredible strength of belief in who you are. Let me explain.

Be Wilder

Firstly, I believe the pathway to performance and mastery requires a fundamental belief in who I am as a person. *'Who is Hanny when she is not an athlete or out running?'*

It is vital to be able to answer this question for yourself, and to understand the values by which you stand – to know how to hold yourself strong should injury manifest or setbacks hit.

I didn't recognise this until I turned 30. One day I woke up and thought, 'I'm not sure I know who Hanny is.' I identified myself as a runner but the scary thought was: 'What happens if I can no longer run?' This set me on a journey to understanding the real Hanny, to identifying her values, fears, strengths, weaknesses and opportunities. Nearing the end of this process, I have found a deeper sense of resilience, self-empowerment, and a confidence in myself that I didn't know I had. In other words, I found my feet. I call this depth of understanding 'Being Wilder'.

Play Wilder

I hope that you have picked up this book because you are also looking to find more joy from this sport of trail running that you have come to love. It is vital that a desire to have fun is at the heart of the decisions you make and the actions you take. Therefore, once you know who you are and what makes you 'you', then it is time to honestly begin to identify what you love. Take away the influence of others, and try not to let FOMO (Fear of Missing Out) guide your decisions. What do you love? If one of your answers does not involve trail running then use a little caution. A love of running wilder on the trails is vital to longevity in the sport and to optimising your abilities.

I call this playfulness and understanding of what makes you tick 'Playing Wilder'.

Perform Wilder

If you know how to Be Wilder and to Play Wilder, only then are you ready to truly perform at your greatest ability. It is vital to arm yourself with knowledge, skills and self-awareness of your uniqueness as an athlete. This depth of understanding will come not only from your ability to read widely, ask questions and learn from others, but also from your ability to get your hands dirty and learn from your own experiences. There is no better place to learn than from failures! When you finally stand on the start line of your chosen grand adventure you will be self-empowered, ready to play hard, and willing to strive for success. That is, you will be ready to 'Perform Wilder'!

The three secrets to success

Three key elements will provide confidence in your abilities, especially at races or on wild adventures:

1. **Knowledge**: How well you know the course you wish to run and what you are in for.

2. **Nutrition and hydration**: How well you understand and have practised your fuelling strategies for your chosen goal, including problem solving when things get tough.

3. **Consistency in training**: How successfully you executed consistent days and weeks of training to create a long, coherent period of preparation.

The common approaches

I have found that when adult athletes are underperforming, they often fall into one of three categories.

1. One-hit wonders

The athletes who grab at their moments of spare time, rushing out the door for a run. They move by feel and 'shoulds'. Their training may be hard or easy, depending on the amount of time they have available. Large or fast bouts of exercise can be followed by numerous rest days until the next session can be squeezed in.

- **Error**: Inconsistent training loads place sudden bouts of shock and stress on the body. These athletes find it hard to produce consistent performances and often experience soft-tissue injuries.

2. Runners

The athletes who love to run but prefer to 'just run'. Training is often at an even intensity – neither hard nor easy.

- **Error:** Leads to frequently running in the 'plod zone', limiting their potential, come race day. These athletes can feel frustrated when race performance does not match their training volumes.

3. Harder is better

These athletes push for rapid strength and speed improvements. Most sessions are conducted at higher intensities or larger volumes, with minimal thought given to rest or recovery periods unless injury niggles suggest otherwise. Gym sessions are tough, swims are tough, and runs are long and tough.

- **Error:** Insufficient planned recovery makes this training strategy unsustainable over a longer period of time. These athletes frequently experience niggles.

If the key to excellent preparation is the consistency of your training, then any of these errors can limit you from reaching your true potential when it comes time to excel.

2. Stress, stressors and smart training

LIFE CAN FEEL FULL. OH SO FULL! OUR MODERN LIFE-styles are full of stressors. Balancing our daily responsibilities with our competing desires for health, adventure and playfulness is a fine juggling act. It is easy to find ourselves with the continuous sensation of running away from a tiger – to the detriment of our health, energy and ability to strive for excellence. Trust me, I have run away from my fair share of 'tigers'!

During nine years in the coaching industry and twenty years in the elite sports environment, I have fostered a fascination with how to train for optimal performance without experiencing chronically heightened stress loads. I wish to avoid that sensation of, 'I am just keeping in front of the tiger!' Experience has shown me that the greatest challenge for us as adults is to balance our aspirations against complex working, personal and social lifestyles.

Sports science research does not really provide solutions as most of the research has been conducted on elite and professional athletes who often lead very different lifestyles. It was quite a contrast when I lived and worked at the Australian Institute of Sport in 2011–12. There, the athletes had a fantastic support network assisting them in their pathway towards their goals. They would often, albeit not always, train and race under reduced external demands, such as through part-time employment or studies.

I found more and more frequently that many well-documented training theories are hard to implement with adults without triggering an overtraining complex, leading to unnecessary injury niggles, sickness, suppressed mood and more. Structuring training in the format of *a wave* has become my solution to helping adults. I have found that over the seven years I have been assisting individuals to implement *Wave Training*, it has led to exceptionally low injury and overtraining rates.

To understand the significance of Wave Training and how it can assist you with your goals, it is imperative to first understand the impact and risks associated with stress.

Stress: The fight-or-flight response

Stress is the body's reaction to a physical, mental or emotional change in our normal, balanced state. In an ideal world, our body would deal with all stressors one at a time via the *fight-or-flight response*. Our body's fight-or-flight response activates the nervous and hormonal systems when the stressor (the 'tiger') pounds towards us. The nervous and hormonal systems ensure that the heart and breathing rates accelerate; blood is relocated to the heart, lungs and muscles for movement; functioning of the gastrointestinal tract is inhibited; and mobilisation of energy sources occurs. Then, once the danger is dealt with, we return to our steady state.

However, there are two interesting things about the human stress response:

1. It is a one-size-fits-all mechanism. That is, the body cannot distinguish between different stressors, whether they derive from your workplace, family life, pain, other discomforts, environmental inputs, diet or even exercise.

2. Stressors compound. The accumulation of these individual stressors can lead to a chronic stress response in which the body remains in a heightened state of stress-induced arousal.

Hormones and stress: A tight link

The stress response is controlled by both the nervous and hormonal systems of our bodies. However, I have found that one of the most interesting impacts that stress has on us, especially as athletes, is how it affects our hormonal system. To understand the significance of stress on our hormones, we need to understand the incredible role our hormones are playing at every minute of the day. They help us to:

- maintain a feeling of balance

- feel recovered from training and daily activities

- feel empathetic

- wake up feeling restored

- maintain alertness during the day

- feel emotionally stable

- restore and maintain the musculoskeletal system

- sustain sensuality.

Healthy hormone function relies on *pregnenolone*, our 'master hormone'. Pregnenolone is critical for the production of:

- sex hormones – especially *oestrogen*, *progesterone* and *testosterone*

- stress response hormones – especially *cortisol*, but also *adrenalin* and *noradrenalin*.

Each of these hormones is found in both females and males. However, oestrogen and progesterone are found in substantially higher amounts in women, while testosterone and *growth hormone* are found in significantly higher amounts in males.

Oestrogen

Oestrogen has more than 400 functions in the body and is the main female hormone. It shapes the uniqueness of our female bodies and emotions, makes us feel sensual, brings a glow to our skin, moisture to our eyes, fullness to the breasts and clarity to the mind. Importantly, it gives us the feeling of female energy and sensuality.

Progesterone

Progesterone reduces anxiety and has a calming effect on our mood. It helps us to feel happy and calm, increases sleepiness, helps to build and maintain bones, slows the digestive process and prepares a female for pregnancy.

Testosterone and growth hormone

Testosterone and growth hormone are produced by both males and females, although to a much lesser extent in females. Without testosterone, the body's ability to repair musculoskeletal tissue is hindered. Testosterone is the main male hormone, and assists a male to feel masculine and energised, and creates muscle bulk and strength.

Pregnenolone steal

When we are in a calmer state of balance, there should be ample master hormone, pregnenolone. The body should be able to make adequate amounts of our sex hormones, as well as the key stress hormone, cortisol. However, if stressors compound, such as through poor diet, exercise, insufficient sleep, lack of relaxation, and internalisation of emotional stress, we can fatigue our adrenal glands. When this occurs we effectively are entering a chronic state of stress. The need to produce vast quantities of cortisol overrides the production of our sex hormones, an occurrence that has become known as *pregnenolone steal.*

Living with chronic stress

Up until this point, I have inferred that stress is a negative occurrence. However, sometimes it can include positive events, making it harder to recognise the build-up of stress, the onset of pregnenolone steal and the sneaky slippery-dip into chronic stress.

Positive stressors include:

- physical activity

- uplifting family occasions such as becoming a parent, birthdays, school sport or Christmas

- travel and holidays

- empowering work such as presentations, conferences and work travel

- social events.

Negative stressors include:

- physical activity that becomes forced and routine, without taking into account your need to recover – for example, continually harder days of training or heavy effort

- poor diet

- poor sleep routines

- extreme climatic events such as heatwaves

- difficult emotional situations such as family illness or workplace stress.

Accumulating stressors in the context of inadequate physical and mental rest can lead to a chronically activated fight-or-flight response and can disrupt hormonal balance. Degeneration will begin to occur to our body's tissues, increasing our risk of injury and poor wellbeing. These changes include: alterations to sleep-awakening patterns; gut irritability; suppressed appetite; weight changes; agitation accompanied by poor concentration; restlessness; muscle loss; decreasing bone density leading to stress fractures or joint issues; immune suppression; and overall fatigue. Furthermore, if you are finding yourself required to cope with too much stress then you may be at risk of long-term changes to your mind, body and playful spirit. We cover these effects in more detail later in the chapter on Overtraining Syndrome.

LISTEN

Episode #09 Holistic Health and Hormonal Harmony on the Find Your Feet Podcast. This conversation features integrative medical practitioner, Dr Sally Chapman. *hannyallston.com.au/podcast*

---

3. Building your foundations

OVER THE YEARS, I HAVE HAD MY FAIR SHARE OF INJU- ry niggles and major learning curves. As a younger athlete, I always thought that more was better and that my body was tough enough to cope with a mess of speed, volume and strength all thrown in togeth- er. Thankfully none of these niggles ever progressed to serious injuries and I believe that I can truthfully track this back to a series of outstanding coaches who put me on the *safe* track over the years. These were Max Cherry, Barry Magee and Jackie Fairweather (nee Gallagher). As I have progressed into a career in distance running education, I have become in- creasingly aware of their influence on my running and coaching, particularly when it comes to injury prevention.

I will share my own methods as well as those inspired by my coaching mentors. I see a vital need to buf- fer injuries through investing in an aerobic base and through *periodisation*. Periodisation is a training tech- nique which requires cycling through various activ- ities and training loads to avoid over-training. For example, rather than attempting to continually build and build with greater and greater volumes of training, we can use systematic fluctuations in training durations, intensities and activities to allow the body more time to adapt.

LISTEN

Episode #30 After Sacrifices for Performance with Jodie Willett on the Find Your Feet Podcast. This conversation features elite Australian mountain biker and coach, Jodie Willett. *hannyallston.com.au/podcast*

Start with base training

Whether we are just starting out in the sport, are coming back from injury, or are aiming for elite performances, we must all build the largest base of aerobic training that we can. Irrespective of age or distance specialisations, building a substantial aerobic fitness base assists to protect us from injury and to sustain maximum performance abilities. Without this aerobic foundation, and as running speeds and intensity increase closer to races, a myriad of yo-yo performances, injuries and disrupted training can occur. In my latter years as a marathon runner, and without the direction of a coach, I fell into the trap of increasing my anaerobic training to the detriment of my aerobic base. Injury niggles and underperformance ensued.

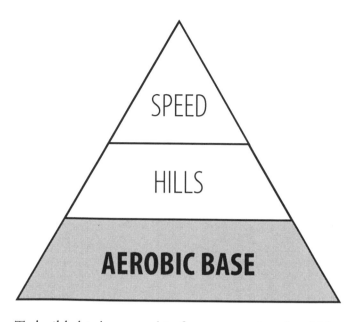

To build this base aerobic fitness, running should be conducted frequently and at intensities low enough for the oxygen intake to adequately meet the energy demands of the working muscles. In practical terms, in a fit athlete this type of running can be maintained for many minutes or hours and focuses on lower heart rates (I find that this is generally between 60% and 80% of your maximum heart rate). If an athlete can easily talk and run at the same time, then they are certainly working in their aerobic training zones as talking is a process that requires oxygen.

I believe that it is better to enjoy shorter, frequent runs to build this fitness, rather than falling into the trap of *one-hit wonder* training, or longer, harder efforts conducted infrequently. It is much harder under this regular style of lower-effort training to develop injuries, and it will only assist you to build strength and speed as your training progresses.

Furthermore, I have found that we can achieve 80–90% of our maximum ability enjoying only base training. That is, if you never find the ability, need or desire to progress into formal hill or speed training, just try to maintain a regular pattern of base training. You will be amazed at what you can still achieve!

Here are some popular types of base training:

- frequent shorter runs at a talking pace

- mid-week longer runs up to 90 minutes in duration at a talking pace

- casual running over hillier terrain

- longer weekend runs and *Missions* (long, adventurous runs) at a talking pace

- *tempo running* at a comfortably-uncomfortable pace. That is, running at an effort at which you can just maintain a conversation. These tempo runs may be uphill.

- longer intervals where you are running at a comfortably-uncomfortable pace, with short jogging recoveries between each. You should never feel a strong production of lactic acid during such intervals.

- hiking, walking and lower intensity cross-training

- lower weight or body weight training in the gym, especially with greater repetitions and little or no recovery between efforts.

If you are waiting to start formal training, are between events or are wondering where to start at all, head out the door for frequent runs, mostly shorter and more achievable, with the occasional longer run or walk to develop your base fitness. You will really set yourself up well to start a more formal training regime.

LISTEN

Episode #19 Base Training with Hanny Allston on the Find Your Feet Podcast. This is a conversation between me and a colleague about the importance of, and strategies behind, optimal base training. *hannyallston.com.au/podcast*

Use hill training to develop strength and fitness

Arthur Lydiard was a famed New Zealand running coach who led many great athletes to Olympic and elite performances. Among his teachings was an avid belief in the importance of periodisation and the individualisation of training programs. This is certainly what attracts me and many others to his coaching principles.

Lydiard strongly advocated that the foundations of training lay in the development of the strong aerobic base, but then following this, he required his athletes to move into a transition phase characterised by hill resistance and leg-speed training. Barry Magee, one of Lydiard's pupils and now a famous New Zealand distance running coach, also bases all of his training on these principles.

The purpose of the transition phase was to continue to maintain the aerobic base but also to strengthen the leg muscles in preparation for the anaerobic training that was soon to follow. Lydiard's hills were not classed as *intervals* like the ones we often carry out here in Australia, but rather bounding, springing and bouncing up the hills to define the muscles and develop the running technique required to run fast. Lydiard's alternative was to conduct this training in a gym setting with a focus on leg strength and *plyometrics*, exercises which assist athletes to build explosive power and enhance strength when moving at speed.

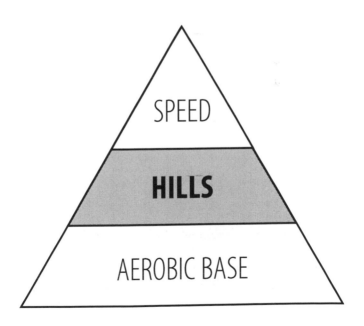

For trail runners, I believe that it is vital to incorporate as much hill training as we can into our programs. Earlier in the training progression, this can by the incorporation of rolling hills into our recovery and easier aerobic runs. Don't shy away from them, as it is difficult to develop injuries running up hills. As your base fitness improves and you find yourself ready for more challenges, begin to work harder on the hills. This could be as simple as running the hills harder or making them longer. Alternatively, you may find yourself ready to start the hill repetitions, as directed in my programs and discussed below.

Here are some popular types of hill training:

- running uphill for long periods

- working harder on the uphill than on the flatter terrain during a run

- uphill intervals such as running strong uphill for a certain duration before turning around, jogging back to the bottom and then climbing uphill harder again

- running on very soft surfaces such as sand

- heavier weight training with greater numbers of repetitions and shorter recoveries

- plyometic strength training

- cycle training, especially when you are out of the saddle and standing on the pedals.

Hills are essential for developing leg strength and are the most efficient way of building on your base fitness. Furthermore, they are the key to developing great running form – when you run poorly up a hill it will only feel even more awful! The only way to become better at hills is to run hills.

I talk about this in coming chapters but I used to have a rule for my athletes that they had to run anything that was uphill but they could walk anything that was flat or downhill. Even a drainage ditch on a long epic uphill could allow you to walk a few steps, so long as you kept running afterwards. This became a sure way of building strength and fitness, and learning to embrace the hills. Make them your secret weapon!

LISTEN

Episode #25 Hill Training and Running Technique with Hanny Allston on the Find Your Feet Podcast. This is a conversation between me and a colleague about the importance of hill training and how to optimise your running technique on the ups and downs. *hannyallston.com.au/podcast*

Speed training comes last

It is imperative that we only embark on the speed once we have undertaken a very strong period of base and hill training. I believe that most athletes are not ready for conducting high speed running such as fast interval training until they have had a period of at least six months of base training. Obviously, there are variations in this rule. For example, an athlete who has been running consistently since a young age will have developed their base fitness over such a long period of time that they can launch into speed training with greater ease. This also applies for someone who has just completed a longer ultra-distance run after a strong build-up of training, and now is transitioning into a shorter distance event. Their previous preparation will have set them up for this transition into fast training.

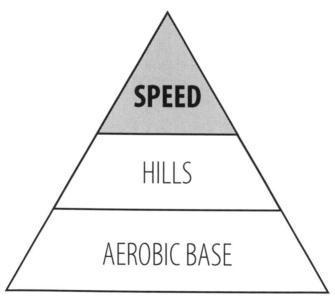

True speed training is really focused on anaerobic training, the style of training that causes your legs to sear and your heart rate to go through the roof. This burning sensation is created by the production of *lactic acid* as your breathing and heart rate struggle to provide enough oxygen to your working muscles.

Here are some popular types of speed training:

- shorter intervals requiring you to run at close to maximum effort

- running when you cannot hold a conversation with anyone

- shorter distance racing such as the 5–21 km flatter, faster events. This includes Parkruns, cross-country and fun runs.

- track athletics training in almost all its forms

- intense power training in the gym, normally with heavier weights, shorter repetitions and longer recovery periods between efforts

- most CrossFit programs, bootcamps and group gym classes requiring you to work at near maximum intensity, especially when they include shorter sprints

- stair efforts.

4. Wave Training: Train smarter

WAVE TRAINING IS MY OWN THEORY AND TERMINOLOGY for a training structure that ebbs and flows in intensity and volume. It is a form of training periodisation to help avoid the symptoms of chronic, heightened stress loads. Acute physical exercise, a potent physical stressor, activates the release of cortisol from the adrenal glands and in turn, the normal stress response. This is absolutely appropriate so long as adequate recovery time follows these bouts of physical activity and we can return to a physical and mental state conducive to recovery. Therefore, in our training we are aiming to create a slowly accumulating load of training that is carefully periodised to avoid over-training.

To achieve this, I construct training in three-week cycles with periods focused on higher intensity and/or volume, followed by periods of rest, recovery and Missions. This occurs as follows:

- **Week 1:** A Moderate Week of quality-focused training. This week should feel doable without stretching you too far. It is often similar to what you have already achieved in previous Hard

Weeks, thereby feeling hard but achievable. As you adjust, what once may have felt really tough should now feel more comfortable and 'doable' amid our busy modern lifestyles.

- **Week 2:** A Hard Week of quality-focused training that builds on what you have achieved in the prior Moderate Week. It should feel challenging but rewarding, with the focus of this week being the hard training days. That is, your easy training days should remain light and focused on recovery, but the hard days should challenge you, pulling you to a new level of performance and mental strength.

- **Week 3:** This week is your Rest Week and should contain approximately 4–5 days of recovery. However, we follow this by my favourite session and the distinguishing feature of my Wave Training Theory... the Mission! The initial period of recovery helps to repair body tissues damaged by training during the previous two quality weeks. When the body is fresh and re-energised we can run stronger, freer and further in our weekend Mission. Fatigue no longer masks our performance in these Missions and instead, they help us to build confidence, and paint an accurate picture of how our preparation is progressing.

The following diagram illustrates the Wave Training progression.

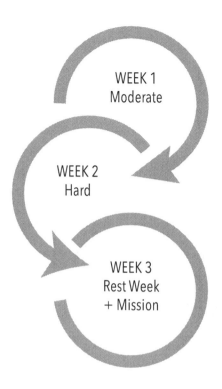

WEEK 1
Moderate

WEEK 2
Hard

WEEK 3
Rest Week
+ Mission

To further highlight how the Wave Training Theory performs, here is an example of how the periodisation of my own training looks.

WEEK	INTENSITY	DETAILS
1	Moderate	The week feels achievable within the stressors of my working lifestyle and I have completed a similar week of training before without 'breaking'. I am focused on the hard days of training this week, ensuring that I recover adequately between sessions.

2	Hard	The week stretches me on my hard days of training and is a progression from last week's Moderate Week. I try to make my hard days of training just a fraction harder than last week, selecting training that takes me closer to where I want to be. However, by the end of the week I am really, really looking forward to my upcoming Rest Week and the ensuing Mission.
3	Rest + Mission	From Monday to Friday, I am enjoying taking life a little slower, ensuring every day of training is helping me feel more recovered and making my toes tingle for the weekend. When the weekend comes around, I am out the door on a Mission! As an example, when I am starting a new training program this Mission is around 3 hours in duration.
4	Moderate	If the last 3-week training cycle felt achievable and didn't stretch me too far, I base this week on my previous Hard Week that occurred during Week 2. This is now my baseline of a 'doable' week. I replicate it as closely as I can while being mindful of how my body is feeling after the previous Mission. This week is important for allowing our training to consolidate.

5	Hard	Once again, I use the hard training days of this week to stretch me, aiming to progress a little beyond last week's Moderate Week. When the end of the week arrives, I know I am stronger than ever but also really looking forward to my upcoming Rest Week and the next big Mission ahead.
6	Rest + Mission	Again, from Monday to Friday, I am enjoying taking life a little slower, ensuring every day of training is focused on recovery and helping me to feel excited for the upcoming weekend. When it arrives, I feel 100% ready for my next Mission, which is longer and more playful than that in Week 3! For example, this Mission can now be 4 hours in duration because I know that my body and mind are ready and willing.
		… and so the pattern continues!

Training terminology

Before I begin explaining how the training unfolds on a daily basis, I would like to highlight some important terminology and principles that I use.

- **Rest Days:** No formal *planned training*

Rest days are a time to unwind and recover. It simply means that we remove the 'shoulds' and try to fill the day with activities that refresh us and allow us to catch up or involve ourselves in life. Kick a soccer ball with the kids, attend a yoga class, read a book, catch up on the bills, sleep in... there are endless opportunities and you will find that the time will fly when you are having fun.

- **Easy Days:** Prepare the body to train

These days are not 'training', but rather help you to mentally and physically prepare for the upcoming training days. Try to be flexible on these days and choose activities that help your body and mind recover and re-energise. This may be a light jog, but non-weight-bearing activities are also excellent forms of recovery on Easy Days.

CLASSIC EASY DAY SESSIONS	
JOGGING	Short, very easy, conversational jogs are fantastic for recovery. However, only choose to jog if your muscles are not carrying too much muscular damage from the previous training. Running too much on damaged muscle fibres will only lead to injury.

CROSS-TRAINING	Cross-training is a wonderful way to aid recovery. However, these sessions must be short, extremely light, and focused on mobility and generating blood flow through fatigued muscles. I like to use swimming and gentle cycling of up to 45 minutes to assist my recovery on easy days.
YOGA & PILATES	Yoga, Pilates and strength training can be great ways to stretch tired limbs, mobilise stiff joints and reactivate sleepy running muscles. I also use these sessions to switch off my mind, sometimes coupling them with a meditation session before bed.

- **Moderate Days**: Volume-building, lower intensity days

    These training days help to build time on your legs. Ideally, for trail runners, the focus should normally be steady aerobic runs. However, if you have injury concerns or like to be more playful, these can be swapped to cross-training, such as cycling or swimming. Independent of your chosen activity, on these days you should be training at an intensity which still allows comfortable conversation *most of the time*. This is a good day for getting out on the trails and loving life!

CLASSIC MODERATE DAY SESSIONS	
AEROBIC RUNNING	Aerobic running is a sustained run at a comfortable talking effort. These runs are the foundation of base training, and provide important transitions from Easy Days to Hard Days. For most of the run, you should feel comfortable and able to converse with a friend, feeling the rhythm and flow of your running. I like to add hills and trails to these runs when I can. Whenever I can, I also try to add one longer run, up to 75% of my standard long run, into the middle of the week. For example, if my standard weekend longer run is around 2 hours during Moderate and Hard weeks, then this run would be around 90 minutes. If I cannot achieve this slightly longer run mid-week, at the height of my training cycle I may aim to complete two shorter runs, one in the morning and one at the end of the day.
CROSS-TRAINING	Cross-training is a wonderful way to get 'heart beats' in the heart. Aerobic swimming, cycling and foundational strength training that doesn't leave you too sore or fatigued are great training sessions on Moderate Days.

- **Hard Days**: The focus is high quality and/or high volume running

    The focus on Hard Days changes depending on what phase of the preparation you are in. Early on in the training cycles, the focus is on base training activities such as tempo running, longer intervals and longer runs. Once your base fitness builds, the focus can shift to hill efforts, hilly tempo runs and hillier long runs.

	CLASSIC HARD DAY SESSIONS
TEMPO RUNS	The concept behind tempo runs is to sustain a comfortably-uncomfortable period of running to build up your aerobic fitness. For example, if the session suggests running a 20–minute tempo, after a warm up you should aim to complete 20 minutes of strong running where you can just hold a conversation with a friend. If you had to keep going for longer you could but only for a short period of time. Cool down afterwards.
LONG RUNS	For most long runs, you should be relatively comfortable *most of the time*. What makes them hard on your body is the number of steps you are taking. You should be able to hold a conversation with a friend *most of the time*, although you may find yourself huffing and puffing up a few hills. If you need a greater challenge, try adding in harder hills by running some uphills at a stronger effort. Long runs are also a great time to practise your trail skills. Mix it up by including a variety of trails, from single tracks to fire trails, roads to parklands. Other than Missions, I try to make sure that my long runs do not exceed 2 hours. I find that when they are longer than this they detract from my ability to recover quickly and perform optimally on my other hard training days. Instead of making them continually longer, I like to add quality to my longer runs.

HILL INTERVALS	The focus of hill intervals is to build strength, stamina and mental toughness. There is no set rule for how hard to push on each effort, but we aim to still run the last hill strongly, albeit with some challenge. The recovery in between should be easy, and usually involves rolling back to the bottom of the hill while practising your downhill technique. Ensure you complete a good warm up and short cool down before and after the intervals.
TIME-TRIALS	Sometimes it is nice to have a sense of how we are progressing. Try to prioritise the time-trials, practising all your race-day strategies including your pre-race nutrition, warm ups and cool downs. During the time-trial, push as hard as you feel confident to push without risking injury or unnecessary setbacks. Ideally, we recover quickly from time-trials so that we can return to training and playing wilder again.
UPHILL 'N' DOWNHILL SESSIONS	Uphill'n'downhill sessions help your body adjust from uphill running to downhill running. You will also learn to run with lactic acid in your system. These sessions are very similar to hill intervals but require you to run more strongly (as per race day) back down the hill after a rest. Once again, pace yourself and try to still be running strongly (albeit with a challenge) in the final efforts.

Day-to-day in Moderate and Hard Weeks

Now that you understand my training terminology, let's look at how the training unfolds on a day-to-day basis. Just like the weekly periodisation mentioned above, the daily training structure should also feel like it ebbs and flows in intensity and volume. Here is an example of how my personal training unfolds.

Week	Week's Intensity	MON	TUES	WED	THUR	FRI	SAT	SUN
1	Mod	Easy	Mod	Hard	Easy	Mod	Hard	Rest
2	Hard	Easy	Mod	Hard	Easy	Mod	Hard	Rest

As you can see, we transition from Easy Days to Moderate Days to Hard Days, adding in a rest day on every seventh day. The purpose of this rotation is to allow the body to recuperate after the challenges of each of the Hard Days. If we allow our Easy Days to be really easy, giving our bodies and minds every opportunity to recover, then we can make the Hard Days really hard. This is where the strength and fitness improvements will come from. That is, we do less on some days to do more on others!

Day-to-day in Rest Weeks

Rest Weeks are critical for the recuperation of the body. We can only generate strength and improvements when the micro muscle tears created by training are allowed to heal. I structure this recovery phase into the 4–5 days leading up to a Mission. This removes so much risk in your training. By factoring in this recovery, you remove the risk of taking thousands of steps on damaged body tissue. This significantly reduces the risk of overuse injuries and excessive fatigue, which often occur following long runs.

The prolonged Rest Week allows us to substantially increase the volume of the Mission each three-week cycle, without negatively affecting our health and ability to perform in the quality training sessions.

Finally, and perhaps most importantly, after a rest you should be eagerly awaiting these Missions, jumping out of your skin and excelling throughout. From now on, you will enter a Mission well prepared and secure in the knowledge that the upcoming big effort will build confidence without risking setting you back in your training.

Here is an example of how my recovery weeks can look.

Week	Week's Intensity	MON	TUES	WED	THUR	FRI	SAT	SUN
3	Rest + Mission	Easy	Easy	Mod	Easy	Rest	Mission	Rest

Here are my final tips on recovering before the Mission:

- Leave Rest Weeks relatively free and flexible.

- Ask yourself every day, 'What do I need to do today to ensure I am jumping out of my skin for the weekend's Mission?'

- Only include light jogging and other cross-training activities that leave you feeling fully refreshed after the previous training weeks.

- Try to include extra sleep and rest during this period to optimise your recovery.

Missions

I believe that the secret to standing confidently on a start line comes from the accomplishment of successful Missions. A Mission is a long, adventurous run conducted every third week of the training cycle. During this run you can trial everything, from how you carry your mandatory gear through to the nutrition, hydration, blister prevention, shoe choices and race-day strategies you employ. Because you have rested in the lead-up to the Mission, fatigue no longer masks your performance or the success of your strategies, especially your nutrition and emotional resilience.

Here are some additional tips for your Missions:

- As the Missions only come around every three weeks, they should become a highlight of each training cycle. Spice it up by going somewhere new – explore!

- Plan ahead so they are fun and take you somewhere new and exciting. On the day, practise everything. Carry most of your mandatory gear. Practise your fuelling and hydration strategy. Experiment with how to stay relaxed and upbeat when the going gets tougher.

- Aim to achieve 80% relaxed running and a minimum of 20% walking. Walk more if you need to. In longer trail running races and adventures, many people have to walk some of the time, and it is important to prepare your body for this variation in load and muscle activity.

- If possible, add in lots of hills and some other challenges, such as stairs.

- Think about whether you need to include night trail-running practice.

Wave Training Theory in action

I would now like to show you a practical example of how my Wave Training Theory looks in real life. To do this, I am going to show you a 9-week training block that I used at the beginning of my preparation for my Ultra-Trail Australia 100 km event in 2017. It is important to note that the focus of this block was Base Training and I already had a substantial fitness base behind me.

Wk	Week's Intensity	MON	TUES	WED	THUR	FRI	SAT	SUN
1	Moderate	30 min light jog	45 min aerobic run followed by 45 min body-weight strength session	15 min spent activating running muscles then 1 hour aerobic run including a 20 min Tempo Run	Easy swim followed by a stretch	45 min aerobic run followed by 45 min body-weight strength session	100 min longer run on hillier trails	REST
2	Hard	30 min light jog	75 min aerobic run then later in day a 45 min body-weight strength session	15 min spent activating running muscles then 1 hour aerobic run including a 25 min Tempo Run over hills	Easy swim followed by a stretch	45 min aerobic run followed by 45 min body-weight strength session	110 min longer run on hillier trails	REST
3	Rest + Mission	Easy swim	30 min light jog	45 min aerobic run	Yoga	Rest	3 hour Mission exploring new trails	REST
4	Moderate	Easy swim	45 min light jog	15 min spent activating running muscles then 1 hour aerobic run including a 25 min Tempo Run over hills	Yoga	45 min aerobic run followed by 45 min body-weight strength session	110 min longer run on hillier trails	REST

5	Hard	30 min light jog followed by a short, easy swim	75 min aerobic run then later in day a 45 min body-weight strength session	15 min spent activating running muscles then 1 hour aerobic run including 3 x 10 min Tempo Running over hills	Yoga	45 min aerobic run followed by 45 min body-weight strength session	110 min longer run on hillier trails, including 20 min of Tempo running in the middle	REST
6	Rest + Mission	Easy swim	30 min light jog	45 min aerobic run	Yoga	Rest	4 hour Mission exploring new trails	REST
7	Moderate	Yoga	30 min light jog followed by aerobic swim	15 min spent activating running muscles then 1 hour aerobic run including 30 min Tempo Running over hills	Easy swim	60 min aerobic run followed by 45 min body-weight strength session	110 min longer run on hillier trails	REST
8	Hard	30 min light jog followed by easy swim	90 min aerobic run	60 min aerobic run but running all the hills really strongly	Yoga	60 min aerobic run followed by 45 min body-weight strength session	120 min longer run on hillier trails (NB. This is the longest run I will do other than my future Missions. From here on I will add quantity not quality in Moderate and Hard Weeks)	REST
9	Rest + Mission	Easy swim	30 min light jog	45 min aerobic run	Yoga	Rest	4.5 hour Mission exploring new trails	REST

5. The Find Your Feet Training Tool

THERE IS NOTHING WORSE THAN FEELING TRAPPED IN an endless training plan, generically written and with little direction to make it your own. Gone are the days of tearing a one-stop-shop training planner out of a magazine and trying to implement it into your unique lifestyle. That really is like trying to jam a square peg in a round hole. You are unique with your own needs, capabilities, hobbies and demands. You need to be in the driver's seat and feel like you are cruising in the direction of your own dreams.

That's why I have a developed the following tool. I sincerely hope that you will have a go at completing it. Alternatively, grab a blank piece of paper, a pen and copy the template I am about to give to you. Fill it in and stick it on the fridge. For if this is the only thing that you do towards your training, I can assure you that it will be the best utilisation of your precious time and an invaluable learning opportunity.

The idea behind this tool is to help you identify all the activities that you currently enjoy and participate in, as well as all the fringe ideas that have popped into your head but you are not sure what to do with them. These may have arisen from talking with friends, reading magazines, your own research and past experiences – perhaps under the guidance of other coaches. We are then going to work out where they fit into your different days of training. That is, we are going to identify whether they constitute rest activities, Easy Days, Moderate Days or Hard Days of training. There will also be a bucket list for all the Missions that you wish to embark on during the next phase of your training, hopefully whetting your appetite for all the adventures that you can enjoy during the training for your chosen event.

Instructions

1. Find a pen and quiet place.

2. Follow the template to create a table containing four columns.

3. Start by listing under the heading REST DAYS all of the activities that you would love to potentially do on these days. Remember that rest days refer to days when you have *no formal, planned training*. That is, these are activities that help you to feel rested and more recovered. These can be great days for family or social time, personal downtime, passive recovery activities such as massages, or other hobbies such as gardening, art, drawing or throwing the Frisbee to the dog.

4. Next, begin to think about what activities you currently love to do or would wish to do on Easy Days of training. Remember that Easy Days refer

to days that help to *prepare the body to train.* That is, these activities are easy by nature and help you to feel raring to go for the upcoming training days. You should feel uplifted and invigorated, and really enjoy these activities. Hopefully they can help to fill your energy tank as well as create potential social outlets in your training. Jot all these ideas under the heading EASY DAYS. Some examples have been provided in the table to assist you.

5. Now move onto the Moderate Days; those that help to *put time in the legs or heart beats in the heart.* These days are neither hard nor easy, but rather those days which are 'just exercising'. They are most effective when they are specific to the sport that you are competing in. Moderate Days are well suited to clocking up some extra mid-week mileage to boost your fitness. Therefore, think about all the activities or routes that you love to run or exercise over that may constitute Moderate Days. For individuals capable of running or exercising more than once in a day, these are excellent days for incorporating two training sessions. For example, you may wish to do one 90-minute run or you may wish to do a shorter 45-minute run followed by a 45-minute casual swim. Moderate Days rarely incorporate higher intensity training such as intervals. Therefore, have a go at noting down all the activities that you would enjoy participating in on Moderate Days, noting these under the heading MODERATE DAYS.

6. Here comes the trickier task. Have you had sessions that you have previously enjoyed on Hard Days, such as a particular tempo run, a hill session, or a time-trial? This column is where you can jot down all the higher intensity OR longer duration training. All activities that may be longer and harder must be supported by adequate recovery. Examples of sessions that constitute Hard Days of training are interval training, tempo running, hill repetitions, longer runs, and hard cross-training. Some strength training may also fall into hard training. However, it is important that these days are as exercise-specific as can be, according to your goal. That is, if you wish to run, then, if possible, these days should directly relate to running.

7. Finally, where have you always dreamt of exploring? Who would you like to go with or what makes your toes tingle? Under the heading MISSIONS, write down all of these ideas. Maybe make a note of how far Missions might be in either duration or distance, so that you can slot them into the appropriate place in the training planner.

Now that this template has been filled in, you can use it to modify training planners such as those available on my website, slotting in activities as you wish into the relevant day's training. For example, if I have suggested to you to go for an easy jog on a Tuesday and you are lacking the mojo for it or the rain is falling heavily, blurring your enjoyment, head to the plan on your fridge and consider what you could substitute this easy run with. Wow, suddenly yoga has your toes tingling and reminds you that you haven't stretched or practised relaxation for a while? There you go! You have an activity most suitable to you on this day. Perhaps you have begun trialling coaching yourself but you miss running with your group of friends? No problems! Head to the fridge and work out which days running with your friends suits you best, slotting this into the training planner when it suits you.

Here is an afterword on this concept. Despite your best intentions, following a training planner might simply not work for you. That is absolutely no problem! Keep this template stuck to your fridge. Add to it. Modify it. Things change and what was once a Hard Day's training for you may now have become a Moderate Day. After a period of rest, things that were once hard for you may now become easy. Your knowledge also changes. If you read or learn about a new exercise or session that excites you, add it to your list. Then, all you have to do is rotate from one training day to the next to the next, as show in the example below.

Mon	Tue	Wed	Thu	Fri	Sat	Sun
Easy	Mod	Hard	Easy	Mod	Hard	Rest

MY SMART TRAINING GUIDE

	REST DAYS	EASY DAYS	MODERATE DAYS	HARD DAYS	MISSIONS
Examples...	Walking to work Gardening Relaxation yoga Family activities	Walking Yoga Pilates Easy swimming Surfing Cycle commuting Jogging with Jenny Climbing	'Just running' Mid-week longer runs up to 90 mins Cycling Swimming Two jogs in one day Running to work with pack Running with Matt	Tempo runs Hill intervals Parkrun Fun runs Running with George Squad training Longer uphill run	Running the Freycinet Circuit (29 km) Exploring the Tarkine Coastline (approx. 5 hrs run/hike) Japan Running Tour (Sept – 6 days)
ACTIVITIES					

Further tips

- **Duration not distance:** In these planners, training volumes are measured by duration not distance. Time is a greater measure of training as it allows us to account for additional or incidental exercise such as strength training, cross-training or actively commuting to work. Furthermore, a 20 km run on hilly trails is a very different training load to a 20 km run on the road!

- **More is not better:** It is most appropriate to measure your training in terms of time rather than kilometres. For example, a quicker athlete may complete 12 km in the course of a 60 minute run while a slower athlete may only complete 8 km. But you have still completed a 60 minute *load* of training. I don't believe slower athletes need to think about going further simply because they fear being out there longer on race day. A higher training load could lead to unnecessary injuries or overtraining symptoms, especially given that we all lead busy modern lifestyles that are less conducive to recovery.

- **Quality not quantity:** Do not solely measure your training by volume, but also by the quality and intensity of training. For example, a really hard week is not just a bigger volume week. In fact, it may be a lower volume week but with tougher quality training sessions or altitude gains in your runs.

- **Cross-training:** Reserve your quality training days for your running, unless you are returning from injury or using that form of cross-training for a specific purpose, such as to aid recovery.

- **Stay strong:** It is important to always be developing and building upon your strength. Make sure you utilise professionals to assist you with this. Frequent shorter strength sessions are more achievable and often more effective than infrequent, longer strength sessions.

- **Don't over-race:** Trying to complete too many races can impact the consistency of your training due to the recovery required. Adding one or two less important events can help you to practise your race day strategies and build confidence. However, allow one-week recovery for every 10 km you race at absolute maximum intensity. That is, a marathon at full effort will require approximately four weeks to be back at full training.

- **Stop early:** If you feel the onset of an injury niggle or sickness, pause your training. Take some extra rest and seek advice. If you have only taken a short break, ignore skipped sessions and just jump back into your plans. If you have been out for longer than 3–4 weeks, return to aerobic base training. Consolidate your base before you begin adding in harder hill or interval sessions again.

Adding races

Races can add huge value to your preparation as they can provide a gauge of where you are at and how your racing strategies are working for you. However, they can also provide a disruption to the consistency of your training. Avoid over-racing. If you do choose to enter an event and use one of my training planners available on my website, here is how I would recommend adjusting these planners:

- In the planner, add any races or extra Missions that you have planned – highlight these in yellow so they are obvious.

- Plan a recovery week before the event. Treat this week like your normal week before a Mission but err strongly on the side of recovery. Add some short 1 min efforts (for example, 6–8 x 1 min Hard/Easy Efforts) a few days out from the race to help you sharpen up. A Hard Effort is an effort which gets your leg speed, heart rate and breathing rate up. I like to think of this as 'blowing out the cobwebs'. Jog or walk very easily between the Hard Efforts to allow yourself to recover.

- After the race, allow adequate recovery. For every 10 km you race at absolute maximum intensity you will require one week of recovery. That is, a hard 45 km race will require approximately four weeks until you can be back at full training. If you participate in an event at a Hard training effort without pushing into the highly uncomfortable zone, allow half a week's recovery for every

10 km. That is, a 21 km race will require approximately one week of active and passive recovery before you embark on full training.

6. Running technique

As I OPEN MY EYES MORE AND MORE TO THE WORLD of running I am continually amazed by how complicated the sport is. The actual *act* of running and how each individual sequence of limb movements comes together to carry us smoothly forwards is more attuned to ballet dancing than it is to anything else. Where we place our feet, the landing point, the subtle shifting of our weight and the counterbalances we put in place are all unconscious things that keep us in a state of running harmony. Further to this, the ground isn't always flat nor the surface we are running on smooth. And what happens if we need to accelerate or decelerate? Go uphill or downhill? Or even crash through the bush with a map in our hand? Imagine that!

LISTEN

Episode #25 Hill Training and Running Technique with Hanny Allston on the Find Your Feet Podcast. This is a conversation between me and a colleague about the importance of hill training and how to optimise your running technique on the ups and downs. *hannyallston.com.au/podcast*

Energy sources

To run, we need to utilise energy to move us forward. There are two types of energy at our disposal.

1. The first is the energy that we hold within our bodies, stored as glycogen or fat. Protein can also be used but is our body's least preferred source of fuel.

2. The second is gravity, our free energy source.

Flat running

When we run on flat surfaces, our propulsion comes from not only the forces we apply to the ground through our foot strike, but also our ability to harness the force of gravity. If we are to move in a forwards direction, these forces must overcome the braking forces that are opposing us.

Propulsive Force + Gravity > Braking Force

The greatest opposing force that we have is the braking force we generate when our foot hits the ground. There are other opposing forces such as wind resistance and how much lateral movement we get from our running style. However, where our foot strikes makes a considerable difference.

It has been frequently shown that if our foot lands directly under our centre of mass, then we have a lower braking force than if it lands out in front of us. Further to this, if our torso is gently pressing forward and giving us the appearance of a very slight lean then we are more likely to have our feet landing under our centre of mass. In this position, we are also tapping into the energy of gravity that will help to move us forward, thereby reducing the amount of energy we have to put in.

Interestingly, a lot of our metabolic energy is expended simply to maintain the vertical forces required to support our body weight. This is far greater than the energy expended to propel us forwards.

Therefore, to run fast on the flat we want to:

- shift our body posture forward so that we can utilise the energy of gravity

- ensure our feet are striking directly under our centre of mass

- reduce any other opposing forces like excessive lateral movements of the arms, loose clothing or head tilting too far backwards

- ensure that we are not carrying too much excess weight (this is why running with water or a pack can also use up a lot more energy)

- ensure that our muscle and liver glycogen stores are fully topped up because, no matter how hard we try, we still have to put in some energy.

Uphill running

When we run uphill it becomes much harder to get our feet under our body. We also tend to want to slouch, which makes us feel heavy. Contrary to what we might think, our braking forces actually reduce by approximately 40%. This is due to the fact that our foot strikes the ground with less force than when we run on the flat. In fact, by the time we are running on a 9% gradient, our ground impact forces are almost negligible.

The reason hill running is so tough is that the *parallel propulsion*, the effort required to move our bodies forward, has to increase dramatically to overcome gravity. For example, on this 9% gradient, parallel forces have to increase by almost 75%. That is a lot of energy!

Therefore, to run faster up hills we need to:

- remain tall, and lean slightly forward to capture some energy from gravity. I call this our *butler posture*.

- increase our leg speed and shorten our stride length to decrease the amount of vertical distance we climb with each step. I liken running uphill to running like a tiny sparrow. When you think your steps are small, make them smaller and quicker! A tip for doing this is to move your arms in tiny swings by the side of your body. Go on, try it! You will notice that it makes your legs move faster.

- activate our glutes (bottom muscles). If you cannot feel your gluteal muscles working then you are relying on smaller, less powerful muscles to activate, especially the hip flexors. This can lead to injuries. If you have trouble activating these muscles, it is imperative that you begin an activation and strength program, preferably provided by your physiotherapist or a strength and conditioning coach.

Cadence

A very important concept when it comes to running with greater ease is *cadence*. Cadence is the number of steps we take per minute. A plethora of studies have looked at the ideal cadence of distance athletes and, surprisingly, irrespective of their event distances, elite athletes in the 400 metres right up to the marathon distance run with a nearly identical cadence of 180 steps per minute.

A cadence slower than this indicates that the body is spending too much time anchored to the ground. This causes a greater loss of energy through the foot into the ground. Runners with a slower cadence tend to feel heavy on their feet and have a noisy footfall. This is quite common among male athletes and when fatigue sets in. For example, have you ever experienced that plodding sensation towards the end of an event or long training run?

To lift your cadence out of the plod zone, shorten your strides and stretch tall into your butler posture. The shorter your stride length, the easier it will be to run at a cadence of 180 steps per minute. Consider this the *marathon technique*. The longer your stride length, the harder it will be to run at the correct cadence. Consider the longer stride the *400 metre technique*.

If you are having trouble making your legs turn faster, try shortening your stride and moving your arms faster. Amazingly, our legs and arms are intimately linked, as mentioned above. I have found it much easier to move my arms faster when my legs are fatigued. Another great way to instigate a quicker footfall is to cheerfully sing 'Row, row, row your boat' to yourself. Surprisingly, this has the correct tempo.

Your cadence should not slow when you run uphill. If anything, it may increase. Therefore, as you begin to run uphill, remember to continually adjust your stride length and maintain your cadence.

Downhills

We are always grateful when we get to the top of a hill and begin the descent. However, often by the time we are halfway down the hill our quads are burning and our knees complaining. Sometimes we can even be surprised by how much energy we feel like we are using up.

When we run downhill our braking forces are dramatically greater than our propulsive forces.

Braking Force > Propulsive Force

In fact, by the time we hurtle down a 9% gradient, our braking forces have increased by a whopping 108%![1] Therefore, even though we have gravity and momentum in our favour, our bodies still have to absorb a huge amount of shock from the impact of downhill running and at the same time apply some energy to overcome these forces.

Further to this, in downhill running our muscles are *contracting eccentrically* (lengthening while under tension) to slow us down and yet we still have to provide some *concentric contraction* (shortening our muscles while generating force). This strange mix of muscle contractions to overcome the huge braking forces guarantees that downhill running is actually quite energy intensive. Research also shows that landing on stiff legs when running downhill causes the braking forces to increase further.

Therefore, to run fast downhill we need to:

- remain tall and even slightly tilting forward. This helps to ensure that your feet do not land too far out in front of you, creating large braking forces.

- soften our knees as much as possible, so our legs are not so stiff and don't jar with every step

- refrain from leaning backwards and placing our feet out in front of us in an effort to slow down. Instead, try to lower your bottom as if you are

---

1   Gottschall, JS and Kram, R 2005, 'Ground reaction forces during downhill and uphill running', *Journal of Biomechanics*, 38, 445–452.

going to sit on a chair, softening your knees as much as possible. You will instantly slow down. When you are in control, raise yourself up as if getting off a chair. Running downhill is very much about soft knees, bobbing up and down, and using your body's height above the ground to slow yourself down. The lower you are (closer to sitting on the chair), the slower you will go. The more upright you are (standing next to the chair) the faster you will go.

- ensure each step starts at the very back edge of our shoe's heel, and rolls through to our forefoot. Imagine that your foot is curved and you are rolling over it, akin to a duck when he walks. This will help reduce the braking force and allow you to roll over your feet rather than slamming them into the ground like a handbrake.

- keep our cadence high. Quick, small steps, especially when the hill is very steep, will help to reduce the likelihood of slipping. The longer your foot remains on the ground and the further it is away from your centre of mass, the higher your chance of skidding.

- strengthen our muscles and practise eccentric loading during strength workouts

- where possible, decrease the amount of excessive weight we are carrying, i.e. unnecessary gear in our pack.

Trail running

Running on rough trails is like a dance. In order to avoid injury and maximise your potential on trails, it is imperative that you practise this style of running and also do not overthink where your feet are landing. This is akin to driving a car. From our experiences of learning to drive, I am sure we recall our parents imploring us never to look at the obstacle we are trying to miss, such as the oncoming vehicle or cyclist, because we are far more likely to hit it. This same theory applies. If you try to position your feet so as to avoid an obstacle, you will almost inevitably end up catching your toes on it or tripping.

So, here are a few tips to help you:

- **Eyes**: When the trail is smooth keep your gaze up and looking ahead. Imagine you are standing on the starting block at a swimming pool, and looking at the water just below the 5 m flags. This is approximately the distance ahead to look when on a trail. When the trail is technical or you are night running, your gaze will naturally move closer in to your feet. However, make sure you are never looking directly down at your feet and trying to avoid the obstacles. Always look up and in the direction of where the trail is leading.

- **Arms**: Keep your arms relaxed and swinging naturally beside you. When the trail is rougher, let them go where they please as this will be helping to keep you upright and balanced. When the trail is smoother, they will naturally tuck in closer to your sides.

- **Posture**: Try to keep upright and tall. I liken this posture to a butler who is ready and eager to serve. That is, he or she is tall, proud and slightly leading forward as if ready to move quickly when called upon.

- **Glutes**: All power and stability starts with the glutes. It is imperative that they are strong and that you can feel them activating all the time. If you cannot, you must start a strength activation program, preferably with advice from a great physiotherapist or strength and conditioning coach.

- **Feet and ankles**: Your choice of footwear makes a huge difference to how you run on trails. When the trail is smooth, a shoe with similar properties to a road shoe will perform very well. When the trail is wet and soggy, a shoe with more grip will give you more traction and confidence. If you have poor stability, especially in the ankle joints, or are known to frequently trip or stumble, a shoe with a lower profile (closer to the ground) will give you more *proprioception* (awareness of where your body is and what it is doing) and allow you to feel and thus respond faster to the obstacles on the trail. Having had a full ankle reconstruction, I always choose trail running shoes which allow me to feel the ground through the sole of the shoe. This gives me excellent ankle stability on the trails.

Stairs

Many trails involve stairs, and it is very likely that at some stage you will come across these in your chosen goal. Like uphill running, stairs are never going to feel easy. However, there is a way to make the stairs feel easier.

Instead of lumbering up stairs, here are some tips to help you master them:

- Whether you are walking or running up stairs, aim to get your leading foot as close to the base of the rising step as possible. I always try to have my foot within an inch or two of the bottom of the next step.

- When you go to step up and over a stair, simply think about how you are lifting your rising foot. Try to avoid thinking about the foot you are still balancing on. If you lift your foot and tip your bodyweight forward, you actually have to move over the step.

- As you lift your foot, think about pressing your hips forward and leaning into the step like a ladder propped against a wall. This will allow gravity to tip you up and over the stair.

With unevenly-spread stairs, if you combine this technique with the *tiny sparrow* uphill running mentioned earlier, taking small, quick steps in between each stair, you will find getting your leading foot close to the bottom of the next stair and lifting your other leg over it much easier.

Hiking

I have observed that we form routines when we are running. One of the most common routines and pitfalls to performance is that when we see a hill or feel we have reached a level of discomfort, we immediately begin to walk even when we are likely still capable of running.

When I first started coaching I had a rule for my athletes: we can only walk on the flat or on downhill gradients; we must always attempt to run the uphills. This is because not only are they easier on the body (as mentioned above), but running uphill is also the fastest way to improve our fitness. However, I recognise that in a racing situation or when enjoying your longer Missions, there comes a point when walking is required to conserve energy.

So, here is how I determine whether it is the time to walk:

• When you first begin to feel discomfort, rather than defaulting to a hike, check in with yourself and see if you can make yourself just 5% more comfortable. Most often when we become fatigued, our stride rate falls, our body posture becomes more slouched and our stride length increases. Therefore, the easiest way to combat this is to shorten your stride and try to stand up taller again.

- If after a short while you are still feeling uncomfortable, check in with yourself once more and see if there is anything else you can do to bring yourself back below the red line. Can you relax your shoulders and slow your breathing rate? Perhaps you may need to consume some quick energy such as a glucose gel? Can you shorten your strides even more?

- If after trying both of the above you are still not comfortable to run ('two strikes'), then this is the time to revert to a hike.

How to hike

There is definitely a technique for how to hike. I used to race in the sport of Skyrunning and once did a race in Italy. On the flatter terrain, I was holding my ground without too much discomfort but as soon as we hit those long, steep mountain climbs... wow, those girls could definitely hike!

The secret to hiking is to maintain a good posture, a sense of determination to move across the ground quickly, and a fast cadence. I like to think about my butler. When I am hiking on the lesser gradient hills, I am a butler on a mission to meet his deadlines. Tall, proud and purposeful. This keeps your core strong, your glutes activated and your lungs and airways open.

For the steeper, longer uphills, tapping into your upper body strength can really help. Using poles can definitely assist you on these climbs as they ensure that you utilise your upper body strength. If you do not use poles, place the palms of your hands on your thighs and push down during each step.

7. Training for hills without hills

MANY TRAIL RUNNING EVENTS HAVE NUMEROUS LONG hills and even stairs. One of the greatest challenges that many runners face is how to prepare for mountainous events when they live in a flat area, such as in many regions in Australia. For instance, some of the runners I am working with live and train in Broome in northern Western Australia. Anything larger than a small sand hill is a very, very long way away. Here are some suggestions for how to prepare for hills without hills.

Run on trails

The sheer nature of trails requires runners to be strong. As you bounce from foot to foot over the uneven surfaces of rocks, roots and sand there is a more holistic activation of your muscles. These are the same muscles that will activate when you run up and down a hill, such as your quadriceps, hamstrings and gluteal muscles. So, if you have the chance to hit the trails and even practise some faster speed endurance work on them, this is a really good training strategy.

'Heavy' fastpacking

Fastpacking is the term used to describe fast hiking. One strategy that I have found highly beneficial for runners preparing for steep events is to load up their running vest pack with lots of weight and set out on a fast hike. The way I load up my pack is to use a 5 or 10 L water bladder or wine cask filled with water. I put this in my vest pack and set off for an hour or two. The muscles required to hike with this weight are similar to those employed to run up and down a hill. Therefore, this can be a really efficient way to get stronger and more resilient.

Uphill treadmill running

While I personally detest running on a treadmill, they occasionally have some usefulness. Conducting a hill interval session on a treadmill can help to replicate the nature of hills. Set the treadmill to an 8-10% incline and carry out a session. You may also like to finish the session off with a short period of time on a stair climber machine.

Flat treadmill running for downhill

Again, desperate times may call for desperate measures, such as running on a flat treadmill. Evidence suggests that running on a flat treadmill has some impact similarities to downhill running. While this strategy may be somewhat useful, be careful not to overdo it.

Get out of the saddle

Standing out of the saddle on a bike or stationary bike is really hard work. Powering down through your quads without sitting on the bike seat activates similar muscles to those you use to run or hike up a steep hill or set of stairs. Building in some out-of-the-saddle work into your training could be really helpful. One suggestion would be to do 10–15 minutes of out-of-the-saddle training before you start a fartlek session (a Swedish training method meaning 'speed play') or tempo run to help simulate what it feels like to run on the flat after you have just climbed a steep hill.

Go for a wander

Walking activates slightly different muscle groups to running. As many trail running adventures can be long and contain many steep challenges, we will likely find ourselves walking at times. The more efficient you are at walking, the less emotionally stressful you will find this activity on race day. It will also help to build strength. Therefore, add in a little fast hiking into your training program.

Take a pilgrimage

If you have the luxury of sneaking a weekend away over summer or the Easter holiday period, then this could be really helpful for your training. Rest a little before travelling somewhere that has luscious hills to play in. After the rest earlier in the week you can go a little bit nuts over the weekend and maximise some time spent in the hills.

Small can be beautiful

Small inclines or stairs should never be overlooked. If all you have time and access to is a small lump in the local park, then just enjoy switching off the brain and running up and down it a zillion times. Just like sand granules on a beach, small things really do add up.

Get strong

See if you can find a local strength guru to give you a hand with a strength program specific to hill running. This can include body weight exercises, skipping, hopping, single leg activities and some weighted gym work. Exercises could include: lunges, squats, dead lifts, single leg drills, gluteal activation work, calf raises and isometric holds, core work and much more. Sometimes you might like to do your strength session before you go for a run so that you can learn to 'run heavy' – the way you might feel after climbing up a large hill on race day.

Get sandy

My last suggestion comes with a little caution… sand. As many of us remember from childhood, running on sand can be somewhat exhausting. Adding a little sand running into your program can help. However, be careful! Sand running places great loads on tendons and soft tissues, such as the Achilles tendon and your hip flexors. Therefore, rather than setting off for an isolated sand dune running session, I recommend incorporating only a little running on sand during a standard session.

While I firmly believe there is no perfect substitute for running on hills, if you find yourself living in a region void of steepness then the above suggestions could help you feel more confident come race day. Start carefully and gently on the path to adding hills because if you have been training on the flatlands for a while you do not want to shock your running legs and risk injury. Be gentle on yourself. While hills may not be your strong point and others might have a few extra gears on the ups, you might be superhuman on the flat!

8. Racing

The psychology of racing

Racing is scary. It is akin to sitting school or university exams all over again. It doesn't matter how much you love the event or the location or the friends you are participating with, it can still be scary. Endurance trail running can be especially scary because it features unforgiving terrains, vast distances, exposure to the elements and even night running. However, I believe what truly makes racing scary is that it is a reflection of you, your preparation, your mental resilience and your ability to manage yourself in the face of discomfort. The expectation and fear is usually stemming from a deep place of internal pressure and desire. Even for elite athletes, it is rarely a reflection of the external pressures.

LISTEN

Episode #28 Adventure and Race Psychology with Hanny Allston on the Find Your Feet Podcast. This is a conversation between me and a colleague about the mental challenges we face to achieve our highest aspirations on wilder trails.
hannyallston.com.au/podcast

Fear

In 2017 I lined up for the 100 km at the Ultra-Trail Australia, an Ultra-Trail World Tour event. This was not my first attempt at this race. Five years earlier I had spontaneously put my name down despite no formal preparations. I had little understanding of what my body needed to accomplish this distance, especially when it came to optimising my nutrition and hydration. Due to a combination of warm temperatures, a naivety that led me to start far too fast, and the eventual realisation that homemade choc-chip cookies are not optimal race food, I bonked at 60 km and withdrew at 75 km. When I signed up again in 2017 I knew that I did so to put this demon to bed – to utilise my newfound knowledge and fitness to slay the 100 km dragon once and for all.

Standing on the 2017 start line, I was fit. Really fit. In January of that year I had completed an unsupported traverse of the 95 km South Coast Track of Tasmania with my best friend. I had trained consistently; avoided most niggles; worked at length on developing a stronger sense of self-purpose; changed to a plant-based diet; and a charity mission to Nepal had me leaner and meaner than I had been for a while. Taking all this into account, I should have felt confident. With the rain coming down, darkness still lingering and cold seeping into my bones I was nowhere near confident. I was terrified. Teary, shaky and scanning the crowd for my husband, I wanted to be so, so far away from that chaos.

When the gun started I found myself swept along by the field, moving in silence and as one with the other runners. As road led to trail I found my own rhythm, moving into an empty space in the field, a location that I would retain for at least the next 50 km. In this space I entered a void, like I had raised walls around my thoughts because I was terrified the fear of failure would overwhelm me. I thought I was alone in this suffering. Little did I know I was in fine company.

I survived that 100 km. From the word go, the only race out there was against my own fears. The winner, Lucy, later said she experienced similar feelings at times. We were one and two on the podium, and we had both been experiencing a bucketful of fear out on the course. Many of the athletes whom I had helped did too. One of my athletes nailed this sensation on the head by saying, 'I just didn't emotionally check-in for the race'. In other words, we physically checked in for the race but left our hearts and desire to be there at home.

Through this experience and having been fortunate enough to podcast emotional intelligence researcher, Dr Clive Stack, I have come to learn that fear is simply an indication of something that you need to move beyond, if you have the power to do so. That is, in this scenario, if I was fit enough and prepared enough to complete this 100 km event, then the only way to remove the fear was to get to the finish line. If I was in a great place, pulling out could never be an option, as it would only lead to greater emotional discomforts. If you have ever tried skydiving and experienced the terrifying fear leading up to the jump, and then the incredible freedom you feel as soon as you take this leap, you will know exactly what I am describing.

To race requires you to emotionally check-in, to bring your fighting spirit to the start line. Fear will try to block your path, to tell you that maybe you don't need to do this one, that staying home and going for a jog is probably what you need.

Don't listen! If the body is ready and the skills are there, lace up your shoes and toe the start line, backing yourself 100% of the way. For when you push through the discomfort of fear and feel the freedom of realising your determination meet your goals, there is no greater exhilaration than that. It is priceless and will only give you greater confidence for your next adventure.

The mental rut

It will happen. At some point in some race you will find yourself doubting your willpower and resilience to make it to the finish point. You will feel the negative little buggers creep up on your determination and begin chipping away at your confidence.

Thankfully, there are some simple tips and tricks to help you get through this valley and work your way back up the other side.

- **Refuel yourself**: Almost all negative thinking has an element of low blood sugar levels. Just think back to a time when you haven't eaten for a long while and are trying to make decisions – and worse still, have to be physically active. I admit to suffering from the worst Hangries (Hanny is hungry and angry). However, a banana, cup of tea and square of chocolate will restore me to Happy Hanny within minutes. This same rule applies to distance running. You think you are down and out? Can't work out why you keep catching your toe on everything? Bumped your head? Feel woozy and distracted? Grumpy? Have a large dose of glucose, preferably in the form of a quick-acting glucose gel. You will have your bubbles back in no time, prancing and dancing along the trails.

- **Keep warm but don't overheat**: Feeling too hot or too cold can make your brain think irrationally. Use layers of clothing so that you can easily add or subtract to maintain an even core body temperature.

- **Use the 5% rule**: I love this! When the negative voices set in, check in with yourself and ask, 'How can I make this feel just 5% more comfortable?' I start with nutrition; then increasing my cadence (rate of my feet hitting the ground); then relaxing my shoulders, neck and spine. It is amazing how requesting 5% more of ourselves rather than saying, 'I need to feel better!' can be so, so much more achievable and produce a far more positive outcome. The same can be said for running up-hills, improving your technique, trying to pick up the pace – aim for 5% better and you will likely create an improvement leagues above this.

- **Consider caffeine**: You do not need to be a coffee drinker to enjoy the benefits of a small dose of caffeine. Within minutes of consuming a caffeinated gel, you will be bounding and racing on the trails in no time! Caffeine is a stimulant and therefore not a true energy source. I like the caffeinated gels because you also get a burst of real energy with them.

- **Don't be a stubborn mule**: Stubbornness is a huge hindrance when you are trail running. Beware the 'I'll be right' mentality. Stop! Do something about your mindset now! Feel a blister coming on? Stop and address the issue. Feel low in energy but think you should just push through to the top of the hill? Stop and take a gel. Don't fall into the trap of thinking you should wait for some unknown time in the future. It will likely be too late.

- **Use energy to overcome anxiety**: Anxiety is almost always an energy issue. I have learnt this from my own experiences as well as from guiding guests in the mountains. When your brain begins to imagine the worst-case scenarios, and you begin to feel the jitters in your legs, soul and spirit, have some quick-acting glucose! Reach for the jellybean bag or take a gel. Swirl the sticky substance around in your mouth, helping to activate the glucose pathways of the oral mucosa.

Within minutes you should feel a clarity of mind returning.

- **Get in your bubble:** One of the worst things you can do when you feel yourself falling into a mental rut is to begin hypothesising about the future, or dwelling on the past. What may have already occurred has now happened and cannot be changed. What is ahead of you is not going to change. What can change is what you do right here, right now. Bring yourself back to the moment. How are your energy levels? Are you the right temperature? Is there something that you need to consider to make yourself more comfortable in this moment? Have you seen the view for a while? Should you stop and just take a minute to ask yourself, 'Where else would I really want to be?' I call this state my *Bubble State*. In other words, when you are in the moment, in the here-and-now, you are in the zone. This is definitely the best place to be.

It is inevitable that at some point, one day, you will find yourself confronted with the unexpected. You will be cruising along the trail and suddenly find that your shoelace has snapped. Or that your head torch has run out of juice. Or that you have run low on fluids. The unexpected even happens to the world's greatest athletes. What often makes them a champion is how they deal with these events.

It was thanks to my orienteering days that I learnt about the importance of *What If? Scenarios*. In advance of every major competition I would spend a few hours brainstorming all the unlikely but plausible unexpected incidents that could occur, jotting them all down in my journal. What happens if my compass breaks? What if I sprain my ankle? What if I get lost… or see a competitor… or find myself last… or gosh forbid, winning?

After brainstorming every plausible incident, I would then methodically work through each of these scenarios in my brain, determining if there was anything that I could do now or in the coming days to minimise these events from occurring, or to enhance the way that I dealt with the unexpected when they did occur. For instance, I began to carry a spare compass in my back pocket, worked with a physiotherapist to learn the most bulletproof ankle taping strategy, and carried a glucose gel that I would use whenever I felt myself beginning to make an error. I wrote a few key words on the back of my hand that I would say out loud when I was faced with a distraction, such as hearing commentary or seeing a competitor, and if my shoelace broke I had learnt a quick technique to improvise.

Over time, the likelihood of something occurring that I couldn't instantly deal with diminished, and thanks to this change in approach, I began to feel more and more confident on the start lines of races.

Therefore, what are your danger zones? What incident could potentially occur that might disrupt your rhythm? What do you fear? If you can identify these weaknesses or unexpected occurrences, you have a chance to do something about it.

LISTEN

Episode #10 Ultra-Trail Australia Reflections on the Find Your Feet Podcast. This is a conversation that I had regarding my experience participating in the 100 km event at the 2017 Ultra-Trail Australia. *hannyallston.com.au/podcast*

LISTEN

Episode #11 Listening to Your Emotions on the Find Your Feet Podcast. This is a conversation featuring emotional intelligence researcher and medical practitioner, Dr Clive Stack. *hannyallston.com.au/podcast*

9. Tapering for races

THERE IS CERTAINLY AN ART TO TAPERING FOR RACES – reducing your training load in preparation for race day. To help you to understand your requirements for tapering, it is important to determine how important each race is for you. I like to classify races into three types, A races, B races, and C races.

A RACES	B RACES	C RACES
These races make your entire being tingle. You know in your heart that if nothing else matters, you want to be ready and raring to go on this race day. All your training is focused on getting you fully prepared for this day.	These events provide invaluable learning opportunities and often provide a great lead-in to your event A Race. They should be close enough to the event that they clearly represent how your training has been going to date, but should be far enough out that you can modify and fine-tune your training as required. If the going gets really tough in this event, you should not dig to the very depths of your ability and risk compromising a quick recovery and return to training in preparation for your upcoming A Race.	These events are just great training opportunities and a wonderful way to remind yourself why you love this sport. They are optional extras, a chance to catch up with friends, to explore a new area in a safe way and gain a glimpse of your progression. Before the race, include an easier week of training. Then afterwards, ensure you have a few light rest days so that you are raring to go again. If you prefer training more than racing, you can take or leave C Races. A great training run can easily provide a substitute for these events.
Maximum 2 events per year, preferably around 6 months apart.	Maximum 1 event as part of a lead up to an A Race, preferably 8–12 weeks prior.	Frequent but recommend no more than 3 or 4 per 6-month period.
A comprehensive taper is recommended.	A partial taper is recommended.	A normal recovery week of training is recommended.

When it comes to tapering for major races, everyone will be different. However, most people will begin to taper off their training around two to three weeks out from race day. This involves significantly curbing the volume of your training and beginning to enjoy shorter sessions that can help you to feel lighter, faster and sparkier come race day. This is especially important for A level races. It is recommended to reduce your training volume by about one third to one half of your normal distances, and to try to increase time spent recovering. Passive recovery should include activities such as massages, sleep, good nutrition and general downtime.

If you are preparing for B level races, it is recommended to still reduce the training volume, although perhaps for only 1–1.5 weeks. During this period, it is still important to increase the time spent resting, but it will be helpful to include greater active recovery activities too. The goal of these taper periods is to ensure that you do not enter the race with too much fatigue. Otherwise your results will be masked and can no longer provide you with an accurate picture of how you have been progressing as an athlete, thereby failing to indicate whether changes are required to your future training. It is also important to recover enough that you are not risking injury or illness by entering a race on fatigued muscle fibres and immune system.

Here are some words of encouragement and advice for your next big A Race day:

- You cannot get any fitter now. That work was done long ago. So just relax now and get ready for race day.

- Due to the repair of muscle fibres, you can achieve strong gains in strength during a taper week. As soon as you begin tapering, focus on high-quality nutrition including plenty of vitamins, minerals, fibre, protein and healthy fats. This will help to ensure your muscles are repairing quickly and your immune system is combating any risk of sickness kicking in. Omega 3s are great for helping to reduce any inflammation.

- For the last four days before your event, focus on increasing your carbohydrates. These are necessary for stocking the muscles full of glycogen, the main source of energy for your central nervous system.

- In the last two to three days before the event, make sure you swap to a carbohydrate-rich diet lower in fibre and protein. This will allow you to consume plentiful energy without risking fibre and protein sitting in your digestive tract on race day. During this time, also increase electrolytes (I highly recommend Shotz Electrolyte) so that your fluid and sodium levels are topped up. Be careful to avoid electrolytes with high magnesium levels, as magnesium is the first ingredient in all laxatives!

- Make sure you rest extra hard two to four days out from the race's start. This will help you to focus on good nutrition, hydration, limbering up muscles with a bath or massage, and generally just enjoying the reward for all the hard work you have put in.

- Resting completely the day before the race will make you feel tired and heavy. Instead, aim for one or two 15–20 minute easy jogs to loosen up the muscles. Include some 20 second efforts at a pace slightly quicker than your race effort. This will help to put a spring in your step, combating any effects from travel, work or the general lethargy from tapering.

- On race morning eat a light breakfast! Try to avoid skipping this meal. Two crumpets with honey or a couple of energy bars and a bottle of electrolyte is an ideal pre-race food. However, if concerned, stick to what you know and trust.

- To prevent blisters, try rubbing Vaseline thickly over Fixamol[2] and place on the high-wear areas of your feet. It is readily available in chemists. Use a merino sock over the top – perfect!

---

2   Fixamol, otherwise known as Hypafix, is a white, perforated fabric tape used by athletes under strapping tape to prevent allergic reactions.

10. Travelling to races

Travel is fatiguing and poses many risks to athletes before major events. Airline travel is especially challenging as it increases our risk of sickness, jetlag, suboptimal nutrition and dehydration. If you are looking at travelling to your event, aim to arrive with plenty of time to overcome these challenges.

Here are some simple tips that may help:

- **Consume plenty of fluids, especially electrolytes**: This is especially important if travelling in air-conditioned vehicles or planes, and staying in hotels with air-conditioning. Try to begin this one to two days prior to departure, continuing a constant intake right up until race day. An interesting note on this is that many of the Paralympic athletes whom I worked with at the Australian Institute of Sport in the lead-up to the London games consumed electrolyte on board aircraft. This prevented them needing to use the bathroom too frequently – demonstrating the importance of electrolytes for optimal absorption of fluids.

- **Stay active**: On either side of your travel, incorporate plenty of easy jogs with some short 30 second to 1 minute bursts of higher efforts. Not only will this help the lethargy, it will help to maintain normal hormonal pathways and the functioning of your digestive tract.

- **Use compression socks or stockings**: This can help especially on flights but also during longer periods in vehicles. This will help to prevent the pooling of blood in your feet.

- **When you arrive, lie with your feet up a wall**: Do this for at least 20 minutes, as many times as you can prior to race day. This helps to remove the blood from your lower extremities, returning it to the heart and lungs for optimal re-oxygenation. This is also a great way of reducing your stress hormone, cortisol, in the body. I actually lie with my feet up a wall most evenings before bed.

- **Activate your glutes**: During long sedentary periods our glutes fall asleep. Include some activation activities such as single-leg bridges to ensure they are awake and ready when you do resume exercise. The risk is that injury can occur if our glutes are not functioning optimally.

- **Eat well with lots of fibre**: Fibre helps to retain moisture in our digestive tract, helping us to remain regular. This is especially true during airline travel. On arrival and once your body returns to regular routines, begin to determine the appropriate time for removing this fibre in preparation for race day.

- **Sleep well**: Try to get straight into the time zone. This is really important for both sleep and nutrition cycles. If need be, use an eye mask and ear plugs to help you get to sleep and stay asleep.

11. Overtraining

INDIVIDUALS WHO ARE CONTINUALLY UNDER VOLUN-
tary and involuntary stressors are at high risk of
causing short- or long-term changes to their bodies.
Professionals call this state *Overtraining Syndrome*.
However, I do not limit this state to individuals who
are simply under high training or racing loads, but
also to individuals who are under high work, social
and personal loads with inadequate physical and
mental rest. In some ways it could be called Over-life
Syndrome! It leads to inadequate recovery from training and competitions with an increasing feeling of
being stressed out. It is also important to note that in
this state, we will inadequately repair existing niggles,
thereby leading to more complex injuries.

As mentioned earlier, working adults with complex
family and personal lives will be the most susceptible
to Overtraining Syndrome. It is imperative that you
closely monitor yourself for the signs and symptoms
accordingly. Failure to do so can lead to the most se-
vere version of overtraining which is frequently referred to as *Athlete Burnout*.

Symptoms include:

- alterations to sleep-awakening patterns

- gut irritability and/or suppressed appetite

- weight loss

- agitation with poor concentration

- restlessness

- low mood or increased tendency towards irritability

- reduced storage of glycogen (energy) in the liver and muscles leading to lethargy in training

- inability to build or sustain muscle tissue

- increased frequency in urination

- reduced immunity to common ailments

- generalised lethargy

- musculoskeletal aches or pains

- inability to concentrate on prolonged tasks.

If you are currently feeling or have frequently experienced at least two of the above symptoms over recent weeks and you can clearly see stressors at play in your lifestyle, you may be suffering from Overtraining Syndrome. Caught quickly, these ill feelings can quickly be reversed through adequate mental and physical rest, adapting stressors where possible and altering training loads. If we fail to acknowledge our body's warning signs, this chronic exposure to stress can lead to burnout, depression and a failure to achieve our ambitions.

LISTEN

Episode #30 After Sacrifices for Performance with Jodie Willett on the Find Your Feet Podcast. This is a conversation featuring elite Australian mountain biker and coach, Jodie Willett, as she discusses her experiences with Overtraining Syndrome.
hannyallston.com.au/podcast

Avoiding overtraining syndrome

Often overlooked, rest is a critical component to any training program. There are two forms of rest:

- **Active Recovery** – light physical exercise to enhance blood flow and recovery processes

- **Passive Recovery** – complete cessation of physical exercise to optimise mental, physical and emotional recovery.

Gentle forms of exercise such as easy jogging or cross-training can be a great way for athletes to unwind while still completing mileage. However, without adequate sleep, nutrition, and time away from the running shoes, athletes will put themselves at risk of chronically overreaching, resulting in Athlete Burnout.

I have found, and from my own athletic experiences, that the most at-risk athletes are those that are self-coached. As a self-coached athlete, it becomes hard to look in from the outside at yourself and your training, and to see when the normal has shifted towards abnormal. It becomes difficult to distinguish between natural fatigue and feelings of stress, and those that are atypical. It can also lead you to unjustified thoughts, such as, 'I am not running as well therefore I must not be as fit. I need to train harder!'

A coach can be the person to assist you to avoid overloading by keeping your sport and life in perspective. Nevertheless, at some stage all athletes will find themselves in an overreaching phase of training or intense competition. During these times, athletes are particularly vulnerable to *allostatic loading,* the accumulation of wear and tear on the body and brain from high stressor loading. This can lead to burnout. Ideally, when athletes are faced with times of increased mental demands, such as university exams, the training load should be decreased to compensate.

If you have not done so already, it is imperative that as a self-coached athlete you complete the Smart Training Guide introduced in Chapter 5. This will assist you to remember and implement all the activities which you enjoy for recuperation and which help you to enter a state in which the body and mind can return to a state of optimised recovery.

Recovery activities

Here are some suggestions to guide you towards optimal recovery:

ACTIVE RECOVERY	PASSIVE RECOVERY
Gentle jogging	Massage
Yoga	Chiropractic or physical
Pilates	therapies
Walking	Meditation
Light, non-weight bearing	Sleep
activities such as easy	Reading
swimming	Journaling
Cycle commuting	Creative activities
Kids sports activities	Preparing for the week
Walking in ocean water	ahead
Stretching	Being outside in sunshine

Identifying overtraining and finding support

I have found that the best way to monitor how I am travelling is to keep a training journal. This allows you to identify the signs and symptoms of overtraining, especially the suppressed moods, sleep patterns, body weight and the frequency and severity of niggles as they manifest. For women, I also suggest keeping track of your menstrual cycles and mood using a smartphone app. Any alterations to normal cycles can be indicative of a body struggling to maintain the stressor loads.

If you recognise that you have been in a state of over-training for some time, it may take many weeks or even months for you to return to a healthier place. This will be entirely dependent on how effectively you can foster a recovery state for your body. Reducing the loads a little but otherwise trying to battle-on-through will only prolong the above sensations and continue to manifest in performing below your ability. Therefore, I would recommend continuing exercising but only participating in Rest, Easy or infrequent Moderate activities for only 30–45 minutes per day, and never at the expense of sleep or optimal nutrition, until vitality returns.

There are many psychological interventions utilised in life and sport. Notably, sports psychology has taken on an important role in preventing injury, illness and burnout. Psychologists can introduce athletes to techniques such as breathing control, muscular relaxation, imagery, self-talk and cognitive reprogramming. Modifying training planners to indicate when high-intensity activities such as competitions and examinations are going to occur, then reducing the training intensity during these times, will help to stave off chronically-elevated stress levels. Further to this, integrating other remedial disciplines such as massage, chiropractic and physiotherapy into your routines can also help you to identify when you may be about to tip over the edge.

Away from the training arena, there are many services offered to assist in alleviating stress. Many universities, schools and workplaces provide links to counsellors or life coaches to help individuals find an adequate balance between responsibilities and play.

Taking time out is not a selfish act

Here comes my final word on rest, recovery and overtraining...

It becomes easy to 'should' ourselves into tasks because they are our routines, represent normality, or they are building up around us in to-do lists and emails. But taking time out is not a selfish act and will not affect your productivity or performance. Quite the contrary! Creating space for *you* should be seen as an investment that can reboot your energy and hormonal health, and return playfulness to your lifestyle. After all, would your body really want to enter recovery mode while you are running away from a tiger?

If you don't like the idea of sitting on the couch and doing nothing then take heart. Rest comes in many forms. The ultimate state of repair is when you are asleep, but taking a wander outdoors, reading an uplifting book, sipping coffee with a friend, lying in the grass with your son and staring at the stars... these can all confront the tiger.

But it is also about playing and training smart. Don't turn exercise into a continual stress. Make sure your energy is expended in waves, using the information here and in my training planners to assist you. This is especially important if you are training for events or races. Because if you do play and rest 'smart' then you will be in a much better place to enjoy helping others, live with greater adventure, and maximise your potential.

Therefore, be brave. Take some time out for you! Power down the computer. Turn off the alarm. Head out for a wander. Find a view. And *earth* in wilder surrounds.

LISTEN

Episode #08 Rowing Backwards to Running Forwards on the Find Your Feet Podcast. This is a conversation featuring elite Australian lightweight rower turned distance runner, Hannah Clark. *hannyallston.com.au/podcast*

12. Common injuries

I AM NOT A TRAINED PHYSIOTHERAPIST OR SPORTS physician. However, there are a few highly common injuries that I wish to discuss because when treated efficiently and effectively you will be able to get back onto the trails faster. Prompt, focused treatment can make what can otherwise be a lengthy, frustrating recovery a quick and painless one.

ITB Syndrome: Knee pain

The most common injury that I see among distance runners is Iliotibial Band Syndrome, otherwise known as ITB Syndrome. This injury normally presents suddenly as a sharp digging, knife-like pain in the front or slightly lateral aspect of the knee. It is usually especially painful when walking up or down stairs, when rising off a chair, or when squatting. It is not uncommon for it to flare on the uphills or downhills. The pain is intense and often hard to run through. It can come on in training but it can also suddenly flare up during a long-distance race, even when an athlete has no prior history of knee pain.

The cause of ITB Syndrome is the overuse of the hip flexor muscles, scientifically known as the *tensor fasciae latae* muscle (commonly referred to as the TFL). When an athlete has poor gluteal, or bottom muscle, activation, the TFL muscle kicks into activation. It will work to help you stabilise when your core or hip stability is weak, either through fatigue or lack of activation, and to also generate power, especially when going uphill or up stairs.

The most at-risk individuals for ITB Syndrome are those with the following risk factors:

- long periods of desk or sedentary work

- long periods sitting down such as airline or car travel

- cycling with poor glute activation

- running with poor glute activation and hip stability

- sufferers of lower back pain

- women (we tend to have weaker gluteal muscles and greater hip movement due to our child-bearing capabilities)

- rapidly increased training loading

- strength training heavily focused on squatting and the core without adequate underlying stability.

To prevent ITB Syndrome, it is imperative that the gluteal muscles, both the smaller, deeper muscle fibres as well as the larger gluteus maximus and minimus muscles, are active and strong. If you notice that you do not have a strong-looking bottom with substantial curves, and meet some of the above risk factors, you may be at risk. Therefore, working with a physiotherapist or strength and conditioning coach can help you reduce the likelihood of such complications. Activating your gluteal muscles prior to every run can help to turn them on.

If you are experiencing ITB Syndrome, rest rarely helps. I have found that almost the only fix is a deep dry-needling treatment in my hip flexors combined with stretching of these muscles and a rigid gluteal-strengthening program. Continuing to run up hills is imperative to continue to maintain strong glutes. I have found that trying to roll on the ITB (lateral aspect of the upper leg) using foam rollers does very little to reduce the symptoms as it is not a muscle but rather a fibrous fascia. If anything, foam rolling tends to aggravate the ITB. Therefore, find a great physiotherapist or massage practitioner and begin a rigid course of dry needling, stretching and gluteal activation. Adapt your training accordingly.

Achilles tendonitis

Achilles problems are hugely common among runners, especially runners conducting speed training, or increasing their training or racing volumes. The Achilles tendon connects the calf muscle to the heel bone. *Achilles tendonitis* is a loading issue. You have either increased your load through upping your training or racing mileage too fast, bumped up the speed too quickly, or altered your footwear such as to a low drop shoe. Furthermore, you may be experiencing weak running muscles. Weak glutes or calves can be the problem behind your Achilles tendonitis diagnosis and I would be asking any physiotherapist to check strength in these areas before writing your rehabilitation program.

However, irrespective of strength weaknesses or imbalances, the most important treatment for Achilles tendonitis is to adapt your load. There are three phases of Achilles tendonitis and identifying which one you are in is imperative to generating the right rehabilitation response:

1. **Phase 1 – The acute onset:** This phase is characterised by acute inflammation around or adjacent to the Achilles tendon. It lasts for approximately two weeks. During this phase, the tendon is acutely inflamed and it is imperative to rest. As soon as you feel discomfort in the tendon, stop. Rest and swap to lower loading exercise such as cycling, swimming or walking until you feel no stiffness in the tendon in the morning. If you do adapt quickly to an acute onset of tendonitis, the tendon should settle within the two-week period.

2. **Phase 2 – Grumpy tendon:** This phase is characterised by inflammation or pain of the actual Achilles tendon and can be accompanied by a sharper pain during activity. This phase will last for as long as you let it, and generally takes the same length of time to heal as the time which you allowed it to remain grumpy. That is, if you have been running on a grumpy tendon for a month,

you can expect the tendon to take at least one month, if not more, to heal – so long as you remain religious in executing your treatment protocols. During this phase of the rehabilitation, it is absolutely vital to only load the tendon every 72 hours. Activities like running and your physio exercises are considered a load. In between, swap to low loading activities such as cycling and swimming.

3. **Phase 3 – Chronic Achilles tendonitis**: Don't let it get to this stage! Now the fibres in the tendon are weakening. It can lead to rupture if left untreated. Blood vessels are entering the tendon and the fibres are thickening to try to strengthen the Achilles. This results in less elasticity in the tendon and a greater tendency for further issues. Continuing to monitor your load, avoiding high loading activities less than 72 hours apart, and monitoring for morning stiffness is vital. If you have waited 72 hours and you are still experiencing strong morning stiffness, I would recommend prioritising your physio rehabilitation and going for a swim or ride instead.

Trust me when I say this, Achilles tendonitis is a real pain. The biggest challenge of curing Achilles pain is that the region has very poor blood supply resulting in very slow healing times. My greatest suggestion is to jump on it early and really restrict yourself to the 72 hour rule. Try to avoid the temptation of the 'it will be okay' mentality. Every time you overload it you are just lengthening the time you will be in rehabilitation mode and increasing the chance of the tendon reaching Phase 3.

Do not forget the strength training! If you have a bout of tendonitis, see it as an opportunity to address strength weaknesses or imbalances. After my own battles with this problem, I have found that part of the cure for Achilles pain is to also embark on a regimented strengthening routine of the gluteal muscles and core. My reasoning is that if the glutes are weak, the rest of the leg muscles, including the calf muscles, have to pick up the slack. The calf muscles begin to try to generate power and this quickly leads to calf tightness and Achilles strain. It is important to note that a trail runner should be able to do approximately 25 single leg calf raises in a row. If not, then your calves are lacking the strength required to run efficiently and with good technique.

When the tendon is grumpy, to decrease this discomfort try standing on your toes on one leg while holding onto something for balance. Remain there in this isometric hold for 45 seconds, because this reduces the pain you are feeling in the tendon. Repeat as often as required. I have also found that Chinese herbal patches left on the Achilles tendon for up to 24 hours generate a burning heat sensation and tend to quickly remove the discomfort and swelling. Massage and dry needling therapy on the calf muscles can also help (although avoid dry needle placement anywhere near the tendon itself!).

Finally, after returning to training, avoid all forms of speed training and return to a prolonged period of base training if possible.

Undoubtedly, injury is far and away the most frustrating part of being a runner. It would be a rare athlete that doesn't experience some form of injury or niggle at some point in their running career. If we are confronted with injury, it is imperative that we learn from the setback:

- What happened in the first place that potentially led to this injury?

- How quickly did you begin to notice something going awry?

- How effectively did you initially respond to the setback? Did you allow yourself to pull back and address the niggle straight away or did you think, 'I'll be right', and push on through?

- How effective was your rehab? What would you do next time?

In the face of niggles and injuries, I like to think with my coaching hat on. That is, if this was an athlete whom I was coaching, what would I recommend? Would I support an 'I'll be right' mentality or would I be strictly advocating for prompt rehabilitative action? I find it easier to remove the emotion when I put my coaching hat on.

The most important thing is… do not return to training too quickly. Firstly, try to gently return to a combination of running and walking, mixing it up among other activities such as swimming, cycling, yoga and strength training. Furthermore, don't just go back to your old ways. It is imperative that you adapt your future training approach to the new lessons that your learnt from this setback.

If you have been away from running for some time, the most important thing is to return to base training. Begin with gentle jogging and walking on your chosen running days. As you begin to feel confident and you are certain that you are not compensating in any way while you run, slowly begin to build the running volume until you are back into normal base training. This process may take months, especially for something like Achilles tendonitis. If you have been away from formal running for more than two or three months, a full six to eight month base and strength building phase is likely required to give you a strong buffer from future injury.

Here is an example of a return to running program after an injury:

Day 1	Easy	Low-impact recovery such as a recovery swim, cycle or walk
Day 2	Moderate	30 min glute and rehabilitation exercises THEN 30 min as [2 min walk/1 min jog] x 10
Day 3	Hard	Hard, low-impact cross-training session such as swimming or cycling
Day 4	Easy	Low-impact longer walk

Day 5	Moderate	30 min glute and rehabilitation exercises THEN 36 min as [2 min walk/1 min jog] x 12
Day 6	Hard	If no pain yesterday THEN: Walk 15 min for warm-up; 36 min as [2 min jog/1 min walk] x 12; 15 min walk cool-down
Day 7	Rest	Complete rest or passive recovery activity

Repeat until you can run pain free for 30 continuous minutes and with no ongoing morning stiffness.

From this you can begin to slowly build up the running volume. From a minor setback, I like to consider a six-week gradual return to full training, using pain and morning stiffness as a strong guide. From a more major setback that has lasted more than 2–3 months, I take this process much, much slower, using my cross-training, such as cycling and swimming, as my fitness enhancers until I am absolutely certain I am running risk-free.

It is always important to let our body guide us through injuries. If you feel too much discomfort during or after a session, drop back to low-impact activities for another 24-48 hours until you feel the discomfort settle to a tolerable level as determined by you and your allied health professionals. If it does not, you may be trying to return too early.

13. Older athletes

I AM FREQUENTLY ASKED HOW THE RECOVERY PRO-cess and requirements for rest change in an older athlete. One such correspondent was a remarkable 65-year-old athlete who participated in the Boston marathon. Following the event, he pulled up well except for very stiff hamstring muscles. He explained that even with plenty of therapeutic treatment and stretching, it had still taken him ten weeks to recover. For me, his story raises two questions.

1. Does the ageing process alter the degree of damage that occurs to the body during intensive exercise?

2. Is the rate of recovery for more mature athletes significantly delayed?

The 2017 World Masters Games in Auckland, New Zealand, attracted over 28,000 competitors,[3] highlighting the flourishing interest in maintaining a high level of physical performance throughout the lifespan. Bringing this closer to home, you only have to look around at running events to realise that most of

---

3   Hill, B 2017, 'Masters Games: What you need to know', *New Zealand Herald*, accessed 17 April 2017.

the athletes participating are 'older', by which I mean athletes more than 50 years of age.

Ageing is accompanied by significant declines in physical functioning capacity. Although regular exercise helps to protect against age-related illnesses, our older runners will notice a decrease in performance and, like my correspondent, often a delay in their recovery following higher intensity efforts. So, why does performance decrease with age and what causes the delay in recovery in older athletes?

Unfortunately, a number of physical changes occur as we age that will affect our performance. These include, but are not limited to, changes to skeletal and heart muscles, and altered glycogen uptake and re-synthesis. *Skeletal muscle* is the muscle that generates movement and power as we exercise. Research indicates that older athletes will experience greater damage and fatigue, and that the muscle's ability to repair and adapt is diminished. This could be caused by a decrease in both *muscle capillarisation,* blood flow into the muscles, and *mitochondrial activity*, the energy generators in the muscle. With less blood flow and an inability to produce energy as easily, this could lead older runners to feel more sore and tired, and experience slower recovery from efforts.

However, the good news is that training in older age can impart a protective effect on skeletal muscle, thus delaying these effects. Furthermore, when the body is allowed to recover with effective rest and nutrition, this should lead to adaptations that will prepare the individual for future physical demands and, hopefully, increased performance.

Therefore, a younger and a veteran athlete should rarely progress through the exact same training cycle. The veteran athlete will require longer recovery periods between training efforts than the younger athlete, and this should be accounted for in the training program. Of concern is that continued training without adequate rest actually results in progressive overreaching.

A discussion on recovery would not be complete without mentioning nutrition. Research indicates that older adults may have higher carbohydrate requirements during endurance training and may benefit from the provision of more carbohydrate during exercise. They also will benefit from a combination of carbohydrate and protein-rich foods in the early recovery phase following endurance exercise to maximise glycogen and protein re-synthesis in the muscles. I can find no literature or evidence in my own experiences to suggest that fluid intakes need to differ with increasing age.

Therefore, for runners greater than 50 years of age, here are some suggestions to assist you with your training:

- Increase the duration of recovery following high-intensity efforts.

- Focus on replacing carbohydrates and restoring protein to assist in the muscle repair process.

- If in doubt, err on the side of safety and have an extra rest or recovery day. If required, drop one or more quality or harder sessions each week. Focus on doing one well rather than lots below par.

- Look broadly at the stressors in your life and try to ensure that there are periods of low stress set aside for optimal recovery and relaxation.

Consider racing less to race optimally. Racing will be one of the greatest tests for your recovery.

LISTEN

Episode #20 Lifelong Athleticism on the Find Your Feet Podcast. This is a conversation with Jayn and Yeti Iten, a fascinating insight into the changing mental and physical approach to trail running and racing with ageing. *hannyallston.com.au/podcast*

---

14. Nutrition for endurance performance

THERE IS A WEALTH OF INFORMATION OUT THERE provided to us by the marketing companies of the large sports nutrition and hydration brands. It can be overwhelming, and hard to distinguish good advice from that which may lead to poor or uncomfortable performances. While I recognise everyone is different when it comes to nutritional requirements, here I wish to present some key foundations for how to fuel our mind and body during endurance activities. I believe that if we know the underlying science of sports nutrition then we can begin to make smart decisions when faced with this plethora of choice for nutritional products.

So why is so much of this guidebook dedicated to sports nutrition? The simple answer: because it may be the greatest single investment you make in your trail-running career.

We can expend vast amounts of time and energy to optimise our training – seeking new exercises or pushing the boundaries of training sessions for small gains that add up to enhanced fitness and performance. However, if you have done the work and then do not fuel yourself adequately, all this effort may be in vain. When it comes to maximising performance, I believe that *nutrition & hydration* is the most important piece of the performance puzzle. You could literally be the fittest and strongest athlete in the world. However, if you do not fuel your mind and body effectively then that physical advantage, and all the training that it took to get there, can be almost discounted.

In my early twenties I found myself creeping into the marathon scene. It was never a planned progression. One day I found myself in deep conversation with my coach, Max Cherry. *'You're a marathon runner, Hanny.'* Whatever his justifications, I found myself in full training for 42.2 hard kilometres on the road. Six days a week, for months in a row, Max had us pushing the boundaries of our comfort until we all toed the start line of our local Cadbury Marathon in Hobart, Tasmania.

While I loved the sensation of floating along an open road with physical fitness as my motor, I wish I could turn back the clock and add one thing to that race day, and the many more that followed… an understanding of the importance of sports nutrition. In that first marathon, I swallowed a couple of mouthfuls of a sugary sports drink off an aid station's table, crossing the hilly finish line in a debut time of 2 hours, 47 minutes. Seven months later, with one gel still in my pocket, I crossed the Melbourne Marathon finish line in a personal best time of 2 hours, 40 minutes – a mere three minutes outside the Commonwealth Games qualifying time.

If only I knew then what I know now! Endurance performance requires the optimisation of strong training foundations coupled with fuelling strategies that can realise the capacity of your central nervous system to fuel your musculoskeletal system.

Therefore, to begin this chapter, let us try to understand how successful you are with your current fuelling strategies.

LISTEN

Episode #21 Sports Nutrition & Hydration for Playing Wilder with Hanny Allston on the Find Your Feet Podcast. This is a conversation between me and a colleague about everything related to fuelling and hydrating, both on and prior to races or adventures. *hannyallston.com.au/podcast*

Three classifications of athletes

From substantial observations during races and longer Missions, I believe that there are three classifications of runners:

1. The Blank Stare Runner

The Blank Stare Runner appears to be on a plod march. They will appear not to hear, see, smell or absorb their surroundings, although occasionally they can utter a few words or pull a tight smile. From close up, they appear to have the 'lights off' – the I'm-on-a-mission facade with eyes glazed over. From afar, there is an element of a plod, a trip, a stumble. When I become a Blank Stare Runner, I become stubborn, out of touch with my body's requirements. Behind my blank façade there often lurks a negative mindset.

2. The Weary but Starry Eyed Runner

Long distance trail running is never going to feel easy. There will always be an association with pain and a little suffering. But no matter how physically fatigued, the Weary but Starry Eyed Runner can maintain a smile. While their body may be requesting a plod, their eyes sparkle with the challenge. Despite the fatigue, brief chats and internal encouragement are possible. The lights are on and the mind is willing to see this goal through to the end.

3. The Prancer & Dancer Runner

This runner has the ability to make you forget about how much pain everyone else seems to be in. They trot alongside you, chatting gaily about life and the universe. Their eyes are alight with anticipation. They can be on one challenge and already planning the next one. Their iPhone is readily out and they are happily snapping pictures to capture the memories. They are dancing across the rocks and prancing past others giving praise and a hearty, 'Thank you'.

So, which type of athlete are you? You may fall somewhere in the middle and may shift from one to another at different points of a race or challenge. However, I am sure that looking back at race photos or a training journal will help you identify with some of the above analogies. If this is not possible, ask a friend or someone close to you. Most often these are the individuals with the greatest insight into your ability to fuel yourself optimally. The type of athlete you are is often symptomatic of your nutrition & hydration, or lack thereof.

Race refuelling is about fuelling your brain, not your body

Even for the slimmest athletes, the body has enough adipose tissue (fatty acids) stored to carry you a very, very long way. In endurance activities where the intensity is lower, a reasonably trained athlete should adequately utilise stored fatty acids for locomotive energy.

However, there is one organ in the body that cannot use fatty acids for energy, and that is the brain.

The brain's functional tissues are surrounded by the blood-brain barrier. This is a physical block to protect the organ from harmful intruders and substances. When fatty acid is transported in the body, it is attached to a protein called *albumin*. This creates a molecule too large to pass through the barriers of the brain. Thus, the brain's fuel source is glucose, the simplest molecular form of carbohydrate.

In races, we require input from the central nervous system and brain to keep every other tissue of our body functioning. It drives our breathing, our heart, and our working limb muscles. With an inadequate supply of glucose to the brain, this system starts to slow and will eventually grind to a complete halt.

Feed your brain glucose!

If the brain holds everything together, then we must ensure that it receives an adequate supply of energy in the form of glucose. It is true that we can utilise stored muscle and liver glycogen for conversion into glucose and energy, but these stores are dramatically limited. Therefore, a fuelling strategy for endurance-race day must include simple forms of glucose, the best of which is a *maltodextrin* (pure glucose) gel.

Glucose absorption requires sodium

The absorption of glucose across cellular membranes requires a transporter protein that sits lodged in the cellular membranes. When we begin to exercise, our brain prioritises blood flow to our working muscles, overriding most of the digestive system's needs. This causes the digestive tract processes to slow. However, the body prioritises this glucose transporter and the absorption of glucose over the digestion of fats, proteins, and more complex carbohydrates such as fructose.

Sweating causes a loss of sodium

Sweating causes large losses of sodium, especially over prolonged periods of time such as during endurance races. The amount of sodium varies from person to person and day-to-day, but can be in the vicinity of 1500-2000 mg per 1 L of sweat. No other electrolyte loss comes anywhere near the losses of sodium. This is because most other electrolytes, such as magnesium, are found within body cells. Sodium is an *extracellular molecule* floating freely in the bloodstream, so it incurs the largest electrolyte losses during exercise.

Failing to replace sodium disrupts glucose absorption

If you fail to replace the sodium you are losing, chances are you will not be absorbing the glucose you are trying to ingest; without sodium present, the functioning of the transporter proteins slows. Therefore, the cellular membranes of the digestive tract, working muscles and mitochondria (powerhouses where energy is produced) become impermeable to glucose – they cannot absorb glucose without sodium.

Low sodium and glucose intake affect the brain and central nervous system

If you are trying to rehydrate during races on water alone, you will likely be disrupting the body's ability to absorb nutrition. Furthermore, if you are using a sports drink or electrolyte with inadequate sodium to meet your losses, you may also be disrupting your nutrition intake. Begin to become aware of your sweat losses both in volume and in the salt crusting that can appear on your clothes if you are a heavier sodium sweater. This can be a great guide to judging your losses.

Your athlete classification explained

Hopefully by now you have identified which classification of athlete you most readily fall into. Here are some tips to help you transition to the enviable Prancer & Dancer on the trails.

The Blank Stare Runner

Your central nervous system is seriously affected. In essence, you have become similar to a diabetic with low blood glucose levels. Whatever you are drinking and eating is inadequate to supply sodium and glucose to the transporter pumps in your cellular membranes, and thus, energy to your brain. Try to learn to listen to your central nervous system. Negative thought processes, clumsy feet, feeling cold, dizziness, vertigo, numb feet or hands, or even nausea can all be symptomatic of low glucose levels in the brain. Feed yourself instant forms of glucose along with a higher concentrated sodium electrolyte. If you are nauseous, stop drinking completely and rinse your mouth with glucose such as a gel – the oral mucosa of your mouth has a direct glucose absorption pathway to the brain. If this helps, you can then start to slowly feed yourself simple glucose via gels, glucose-enriched pharmacy jellybeans and glucose tablets.

The Weary but Starry Eyed Runner

Your nutrition and training strategies are strong but likely the quantities need adjusting. Sparkling eyes and alertness suggest that the central nervous system is coping. The physical weariness can be a symptom that further training is required, or it may also be that you need to increase the quantity of glucose and electrolyte replacement. You should also be paying close attention to changes in your central nervous system as the race progresses. If negative thoughts, anxiety, clumsiness or any of the other symptoms above settle in, make sure you increase your glucose and sodium intake. This is especially true if you start to experience cramping.

The Prancer & Dancer Runner

You are nailing it! To run like this, your central nervous system is functioning fully and you are alert enough to absorb your surroundings. Further to this, it appears that your training has prepared you optimally for the challenge you have embarked upon. However, keep an eye on climatic changes throughout the race, as increases in temperature, humidity or wind will alter your evaporative sweat losses. Monitor your thoughts and alertness, with any small changes requiring a top-up of energy.

Hydration for endurance performance

We have all heard that our bodies are comprised of mostly water. A 60 kg individual is composed of around 48 kg of water in which all their body's biochemistry will take place. Water has a number of other functions in the body – evaporative cooling, glycogen storage and maintaining electrolyte balances. The loss of even a small proportion of this fluid (i.e. 2% of body weight) can significantly reduce bodily functions and for athletes, performance. It can also be life threatening. When we consider that this is only 1.2 L in our 60 kg athlete, we begin to realise how significant the process of optimal hydration is.

Evaporative cooling

Weighing around 60 kg, I consume around 0.2 L of oxygen per minute, generating 70 watts of heat output. However, when running at threshold during a *VO2 max test*, my oxygen consumption has been shown to increase by around 16 times and my heat output to rise to 1100 watts. The only way that this heat can be lost rapidly is through evaporative cooling, otherwise known as sweating. Sweating involves the loss of large amounts of fluid from the skin's surface, which is then wicked away by air, resulting in body cooling. In hot conditions, I require around 1.5–2.0 L of sweat to remove this excess heat.

Glycogen storage

Replacing fluid lost through sweat and urine is not the only justification for the importance of hydration. Glycogen or stored muscle carbohydrate is the body's main source of energy. However, fixing 1 g of carbohydrate into the muscles in the form of glycogen requires 3 g of water i.e. a 3:1 ratio of water to carbohydrate. This is one reason why you can often feel thirsty following a carbohydrate-rich meal. With this in mind, fluid is critical during times of recovery and taper. If you are focusing on carb-loading but not drinking adequate amounts you can actually risk pulling extra water from the blood stream into the gastrointestinal tract (*GI tract*). This can result in dehydration. Therefore, fluid is critical for replacing sweat and urine losses, but also for glycogen storage before and after exercise.

Other reasons it's important to remain hydrated

As you heat up, the body begins to enter survival mode. Rather than shunting blood to the working muscles, your blood stream prioritises blood flow to the skin and vital organs. The reduced blood flow to the GI tract makes the digestion of complex drinks and nutrition difficult, and as a result people often begin to experience stomach upsets and nausea. During such periods of stress, your breathing and heart rates will increase, and your general efficiency takes a dramatic nose-dive. Under these additional stressors, your body temperature will start to rise, resulting in stress to the brain. Clarity of thinking will decrease, your ability to assess your body state becomes compromised (runners often complain of feeling cold when they overheat) and you may begin to feel disorientated. All these sound like great things to avoid when racing!

Should I just guzzle water?

When we sweat and excrete urine, we don't just lose fluids but also vital minerals. The main ingredient in sweat is sodium that is lost at a rough rate of 1–2 g per litre.[4] Other minerals lost are calcium, magnesium,

---

4   Griffiths, D 2015, *Sweat. Think. Go Faster: A common sense approach to sports nutrition for endurance athletes*, Australia.

potassium and chloride, although these are generally lost in much, much smaller quantities. Therefore, to replace fluid losses an electrolyte drink is far better than drinking pure water and the focus should turn to sodium.

Why not water?

Are you putting the energy gels in but not receiving the 'kick'? Over prolonged periods of heavy sweating, an individual can lose significant amounts of sodium. The combination of drinking pure water and sweating can cause a dilution of the concentration of sodium in the blood. This can begin to impair many of our normal physiological processes, including, as mentioned above, the transport of fluid and glucose across cellular membranes. That's right, a lack of sodium can inhibit the transport of glucose into the working muscle's cells.

Another good reason for opting for an electrolyte drink is that the use of sodium is known to promote thirst. This is often the reason why pubs serve salty, greasy foods, as it will generate greater drinks sales.

Finally, when electrolytes, particularly sodium, are present in appropriate concentrations, the rate of fluid absorption from the small intestine into the rest of the body is enhanced. This is particularly important to consider when we are racing at intense levels with few possibilities to drink.

What to look for in an electrolyte drink

Always check the ingredients of an electrolyte drink. Sports drinks that are high in simple sugars can be very foreign to a small intestine under stress. In fact, the presence of the sugar that remains dormant in the GI tract can create a net movement of fluid from the blood stream back into the gut, resulting in stomach distress and dehydration.

Therefore, sports drinks based around the medical principles for oral rehydration are preferred. Complexes such as Shotz Electrolyte tablets, when dissolved in adequate water, are proven to initiate rehydration even under the most stressful environments. These beverages contain a high concentration of sodium and only minimal traces of the other elements. This is important because some sports drinks are high in magnesium – which also happens to be the first ingredient in all laxatives! Always read the label, and watch out for tummy-disrupting ingredients.

How much should I drink?

How much fluid you need to consume is dependent on your fitness level, size, *sweat rate* and the weather conditions. Hot, sticky conditions will cause greater fluid losses due to the necessity to lose greater amounts of heat from the skin's surfaces. Conversely, a cool, damp day will require lower fluid quantities to be consumed. The best way to determine how much you should drink is to undertake a *Sweat Rate Test*.

The Sweat Rate Test

The easiest way to measure your sweat rate is to weigh yourself without clothes on before and after you exercise for one hour. Take note of the climatic conditions you were exercising in.

Method:

1. Weigh yourself without clothes on before you head out to train.

2. Conduct one hour of training in as similar conditions to race day as possible i.e. intensity, pace and discipline.

3. After one hour, return home, strip down, thoroughly dry your skin and hair, and then weigh yourself again.

Results

Assuming you did not use the toilet or consume any fluids during exercise, your weight loss is effectively your sweat rate.

1 kg of weight lost = 1 L of fluid lost

If you drank any fluids or used the rest room between the two weight samples, you will need to include both of these estimated weights in your calculations.

- *Add* any fluids consumed to the amount of weight lost.

- *Subtract* from the total weight loss an estimated amount lost from any emergency bathroom stops you may have made.

Hydration: Important considerations

Weather and climatic conditions strongly influence sweat rates. For example, on a cooler overcast morning you will lose less sweat volume than on a hot, humid morning. Therefore, be sure to record the heat, humidity and weather conditions in your sweat test and repeat the test in cool, humid, windy and hot conditions.

Sweat rate also changes with increases in pace and effort. For example, if you monitored your sweat rate for a shorter half marathon race pace and then want to step up to a 50 km or 100 km race that requires a lower effort over a prolonged period of time, you will need to conduct the above tests again to measure your sweat rate in the new effort zone.

In summary, now that you know your sweat rates under different climatic conditions, you now need to develop an understanding of how much fluid replacement your stomach can tolerate. You will never replace the full amount that you lose through sweating, but rather we are aiming to minimise losses and replace as much as your stomach can tolerate. The only way to determine this is to practise, practise, practise!

Cramping

Cramping is almost always a result of sodium loss but can be compounded by a failure to prepare your body through your training for physical demands, such as long downhills during a mountain race. However, if you begin to experience cramping, simply take concentrated sodium in the form of salt tablets (make sure they do not contain any magnesium or you can upset your stomach further), or a very, very concentrated sodium-rich electrolyte drink. The cramping should cease quickly. Following this, ensure that you begin replacing your sodium losses with a quality sodium-rich electrolyte to avoid returning to a cramping state.

Stomach distress – frequent defecating

If you begin to experience the need to frequently stop for a toilet break, you may find that there can be three issues at play:

- **Magnesium loading**: Magnesium is frequently put in electrolyte and sports drinks as there is a common misconception that it is the root cause of cramping. Magnesium is a main ingredient in many laxatives. If you consume such an electrolyte drink over a prolonged period of time then the magnesium can build up through the gut system, causing a laxative effect. Try switching to a more simple, sodium-rich electrolyte solution.

- **Fat, fibre or protein**: None of these are readily absorbed in the gut system during higher intensity physical exertion due to the slowing of these organs to help supply a greater blood flow to your working muscles. The body will more readily absorb glucose-rich foods.

- **Concentrated fructose**: This is a more complex sugar that requires the liver to break it down into simpler glucose molecules. The liver is one of the first organs to slow its functioning when our muscles begin yelling for oxygen during exercise. Concentrated fructose is frequently found in cheaper sugary items containing fruit concentrates, corn syrup or ordinary table sugar, such as lollies, cheap gels and sugary drinks. Try to avoid these where possible.

Stomach distress - vomiting

This is a frustratingly common occurrence in ultra runners. I have found that there is a frequent and poorly understood cause of vomiting in these athletes; water retention in the gut sets off the *vomiting stretch reflex* in our stomachs. Vomiting is normally the evidence of your body trying to empty the fluids that it is struggling to absorb. If you experience or begin to notice a sloshing of fluid in your stomach, there are several things you can consider doing:

- Ensure that you are consuming electrolyte, and at an appropriate concentration for your needs. If this is a frequently occurring problem, try increasing the concentration of sodium in your fluids.

- You may be drinking too much for your needs. We cannot easily stock up on fluids before a race, but rather we need to sip them in accordance with our current needs. Make sure you understand these needs by completing a Sweat Rate Test.

- If the sloshing or nausea begins, stop drinking and eating immediately! Take a strong dose of sodium straight away, preferably in the form of multiple salt tablets. This will act like a big sponge and help to absorb the fluid in your gut system. You should be able to return to gentle sipping of normal fluids once the sensation passes.

- Stress and anxiety sometimes play a huge part, especially if you are fearful of this as a recurring struggle. For some athletes who experience this distress, yoga, meditation and mindful running has helped them to move beyond the distress associated with their nausea.

LISTEN

Episode #04 Fuelling Your Intentions Part 1 on the Find Your Feet Podcast. This is a conversation featuring the founder of Shotz Sports Nutrition Australia and elite athlete nutrition coach, Darryl Griffiths. *hannyallston.com.au/podcast*

LISTEN

Episode #23 Fuelling Your Intentions Part 2 on the Find Your Feet Podcast. This is a conversation featuring the founder of Shotz Sports Nutrition Australia and elite athlete nutrition coach, Darryl Griffiths. *hannyallston.com.au/podcast*

LISTEN

Episode #15 The Trail to UTMB on the Find Your Feet Podcast. This is a conversation featuring Brook Martin, an athlete who has learnt the importance of sustainable training and who has overcome a plethora of nutritional challenges to finish among the world's top athletes at UTMB (the Ultra-Trail du Mont-Blanc). *hannyallston.com.au/podcast*

15. Mandatory gear

HAVING THE RIGHT GEAR WILL REALLY HELP YOUR performance in training, adventures and on race day. In fact, when it comes to running in ugly conditions where you are far outside your comfort zone, it can be life-changing. As my husband once said while we were running in teeming cold rain on a remote Tasmanian peak in new raincoats, 'I should be miserable now. And yet in this raincoat I feel like I could achieve anything!' In this section I will focus on the common race mandatory gear items, highlighting those that are really important.

Key items for trail running

Setting up your trail running equipment and apparel can be an expensive exercise. However, I implore you not to skimp on the following items:

- vest pack

- rain jacket

- footwear

- head torches.

Vest packs

The first time I ran the Overland Track 82 km race I was 19 years old. The day was somewhat soggy and I felt cold right from the start. I used an old daypack that a friend helped me modify to carry water bottles. The pack bounced all day against the skin of my back, water sloshing endlessly like a form of water torture. By the end of the event I had large, welted abrasions across my back. To say I felt miserable was an understatement. I now never underestimate the virtues of a good vest pack and hydration system.

A vest pack is a pack that clasps around your chest without a waistband. This ensures there is no bounce in the pack when you run and helps prevent any chafing or discomfort from the waist strap. There are, and always will be, a plethora of vest packs on the market to choose from.

Here are some considerations for selecting your ideal pack:

- the distances you wish to run

- how much mandatory gear or storage is required

- the hydration capacity required and whether you have access to aid stations

- whether you prefer to drink from bottles (soft flasks) or bladders (reservoirs).

The following table should assist you to choose your vest pack. For this table, we are assuming that you will be required to carry mandatory gear and that there is some support on the trail. We are also assuming that you are a low-to-average sweater. If you know that you are a thirsty runner who perspires profusely, you may require a greater fluid capacity. Furthermore, if you are a larger male with more bulky clothing, you may need to consider giving yourself a little more capacity.

SPECIFICATIONS	RACE OR ADVENTURE DISTANCE				
	<25 KM (TRAIL)	MARATHON (ROAD)	>50 KM (TRAIL)	100 KM (TRAIL)	>100 KM (TRAIL)
Minimum Capacity	3 L	1 L	5–8 L	10–12 L	12 L
Minimum Fluid Capacity	1 L	1 L	2 L	2 L	2 L
Bottles and/or Bladder	Bottles	Bottles	Bottles, or bottles with optional additional bladder	Bottles, or bottles with optional additional bladder	Bottles, or bottles with optional additional bladder

Here is an example of what I have been able to carry in a 3 L vest pack when running, as a Mission, the wild South Coast Track (GPS recorded distance 93 km) in Tasmania:

- hooded rain jacket

- a thermal top and pants

- large dry sack (for river crossings)

- spare socks

- Body Glide anti-chafe balm

- comprehensive first aid kit including space blanket

- 1 L of fluid (I could restock at various points on the trails)

- a mobile phone (for photos)

- a day's worth of running nutrition and electrolyte tablets

- satellite phone plus a radio

- emergency nutrition

- head torch.

A good tip is that if you are using a bottle-only pack but are required to carry more fluids by a race organiser, you can always add another one or two soft flasks into the main compartment of the pack.

Rain jacket

There will soon come a time when you will be on a trail or in a race and it will be wet. Potentially very wet! Having gear that can keep you warm and somewhat dry could become the difference between enjoying yourself and not enjoying yourself, finishing and not finishing. Do not skimp on your rain jacket and thermals as you may be running a very long way in these!

These are the more important considerations when selecting a rain jacket:

- **What is it made of?** Today the technology is incredible. Sadly, while I know this is a broad generalisation, the more expensive the jacket, the better it will likely perform. A minimum requirement for a good waterproof, breathable jacket for trail running is *10,000 mm waterhead*. This is a measurement of how much water can sit on top of the garment's fabric before dripping through. That is, in a heavy downpour, the more waterhead, the more waterproof your jacket will be.

- **Comfort and fit**: Make sure you can freely move your arms and upper body in the rain jacket, including when you have multiple layers underneath. Some athletes also choose to wear their rain jacket over their vest pack. This makes it easier to remove and can also give the jacket a greater life span as your vest pack will not be rubbing on the fabric. I have chosen a fit to wear under my vest pack so that it is not a gaping size when I am using it for other purposes.

- **Pit-zips**: Generally, most rainwear for active adventures will have zippered vents under your arms. However, do not be put off if the jacket does not. In many more expensive garments the fabric has greater breathability and therefore does not require these additional vents. If a jacket has venting holes to allow for heat to be removed, this generally means that the fabric is less breathable. To truly keep me dry, I would prefer a higher-quality garment with less venting and greater breathability in the fabric.

- **Mandatory gear requirements**: Many trail running and ultra-running races require athletes to have a seam-sealed, hooded and breathable rain jacket. What does this mean? This means that the jacket has to have a permanently attached hood, that the jacket allows some airflow when you are sweating in it, and that all the seams in the garment have been taped over (a clear strip of tape to help weld the seams closed).

- **Packability**: If you will be racing, it is beneficial to select a lighter-weight jacket that packs into a small size.

And of course… appearance!

Footwear

Running shoes are designed with two purposes in mind:

1. to protect the feet and body from injury that can result from the repeated impact of striking the ground

2. to assist forward propulsion by gripping the trail or road surface to provide traction, thereby maximising speed.

Trail running shoes have highly specific designs and functionality. They feature a varyingly aggressive sole to provide heightened traction on the trail surface. The design of the shoe's cushioning is normally firmer than a 'normal' road running shoe. Some trail running shoes have *forefoot rock plates* to protect the balls of your feet from sharp objects.

Other important features of trail running shoes are:

- durable fabrics for the shoe's upper

- high grip sole compositions

- often advanced lacing techniques that cannot come undone easily

- occasional addition of waterproof technologies.

Choosing a trail running shoe

There are so many shoes on the market. Here I wish to break down some of the confusion by providing you with a step-by-step method for selecting your shoes.

Step 1: Where do you normally run in your trail running shoe?

The most important consideration when choosing a trail running shoe is what the *predominant* trail surface is going to be:

- **Roads and fire trails**: Grip is less of an issue and a shoe with a smooth tread on its sole is most comfortable.

- **Smooth walking trails:** A shoe with a smoother tread on the sole and a breathable mesh upper is best suited to smooth single tracks or walking trails. Higher levels of cushioning in a shoe are also often best suited to smoother trails, as proprioception, a subconscious perception of our body's movements and position, and balance are less of an issue.

- **Mixed trails:** When running on a mixture of terrains and trails, I prefer to choose a shoe with a smooth tread. There is nothing worse than running in a really aggressive, knobbly shoe on smooth sections of trail.

- **Rocky trails:** When the predominant surface type is rocky terrain, you will require a tread that is not too knobbly as this means you will have less of the shoe's sole on the trail and thus, less grip. I suggest a smoother tread pattern with a durable upper on the shoe to protect against damage from the rocks.

- **Muddy trails:** If the predominant trail surface is wet, mushy trails, you will require a shoe with a deeper tread pattern on the sole of the shoe.

- **Orienteering and off-track:** Shoes suited to this category must have extreme grip and durability suited to harsh terrains. They must also provide enough flexibility in the sole of the shoe and sensitivity to the sole of the foot to enable adequate proprioception when running off-trails.

Step 2: What running shoe are you currently running in?

Next it is important to consider what shoe you have mostly been running in. Try to avoid making massive changes. For example, if you are currently running in a highly-cushioned road running shoe, avoid transitioning straight to a very minimal trail running shoe.

Here are a few things to look for in a shoe. It is best to make sure that you are not making any substantial changes in more than one category if possible.

- **Drop**: This is a measure of the height of the heel above the forefoot. In general, 0–4 mm is considered low; 6–8 mm is moderate; and 9 mm+ is a higher drop. A *low drop* trail running shoe can feel dynamic and light. However, athletes with concerns about aggravating issues such as Achilles tendonitis often prefer a higher drop shoe.

- **Cushion**: This is really an indication of how much protection a shoe provides from the trail and how much 'sponginess' you feel in a shoe. Low cushioning can provide a very dynamic and sensitive feel on the trails, helping to increase your dynamics on rough surfaces and reduce the weight of a shoe. A higher cushion shoe can make longer training and racing miles more comfortable, and suit athletes who are prone to overuse or impact injuries, such as stress fractures.

Step 3: What distance will you use this trail running shoe for?

It is important to consider the distance of the race (or training runs) you are using this shoe for. Some shoes are better suited to long distance trail running races and some are more suited to shorter distance trail running races. If you are selecting a shoe to meet most of your training requirements, or are looking for a shoe for long racing or adventure distances, I believe it is important to select a shoe with more cushion and a higher drop (i.e. > 4–6 mm).

Step 4: Choose your optimal trail running shoe size

When we run longer distances, our feet can swell by up to half a size. Therefore, always err on the side of 'slightly larger' when selecting a shoe, to allow for this foot expansion. The shoe is likely to be the correct size if they feel slightly relaxed. By having this slight bit of space between your toes and the end of the shoe you can help protect your toes from jamming the front of the shoe when running downhills.

Head torches

The most comfortable way to run at night is with a head torch, and to run confidently on trails you will require a torch with a brightness of at least 200 lumens. A brightness any less than this will fail to pick up the definitions in the trail, making you less confident and nimble.

When selecting your head torch, make sure that the torch's housing is very comfortable on your forehead and that when you jump up and down there is no wobble. If the torch shakes on your head it will make the light's beam bounce up and down, casting disconcerting shadows and patches of darkness that can obscure the trail's details. For comfort, I like to use a thin headband under my head torch to protect my forehead.

If you are required to carry a backup light, you will need to weigh up the chances of using it, technicality of the trail, and weight and size of these backup lights when choosing your backup light. I like to make sure that it is one that I can definitely still run by. There would be nothing worse than being stranded on a long night run with a backup light that can barely reveal the trail. For a backup, I prefer a head torch with a brightness of no less than 50 lumens and preferably greater than 100 lumens.

Night running

If your event involves any night running, take plenty of opportunities to run at night. If you have never run at night, start on an easier surface such as a road or fire trail and then build up to the single-width tracks. Running downhill at night is also a skill in itself so try to practise this as much as possible.

Here are my final words of advice when it comes to gear… train with it! Use it and know it!

16. What to do next

IT IS MY GREATEST AMBITION THAT YOU USE THE IN-formation in this book to spur you forwards in the direction of wilder trail running adventures.

- Be brave enough to put yourself in the driver's seat of your own dreams.

- Learn, read, and critique what you are doing, so that each time you run the trails you feel more empowered and prepared.

- As your performance improves, you will find that your ability and desire to Play Wilder grows too.

On my website you will find a growing collection of running-training planners for specific events and distances. The planners are designed to support *The Trail Running Guidebook* by providing customised assistance for your chosen endeavour.

The durations covered by the training plans range from ten weeks up to six months.

They are suitable for anyone of any ability, although the longer distances such as the 100 Miler will assume that you have a strong history of running behind you.

Visit **hannyallston.com.au/training-resources.html** to explore:

1. **EVENT-SPECIFIC PLANS** including Ultra-Trail Australia events, Point to Pinnacle uphill half-marathon, and the Run Larapinta multi-day stage races.

2. **DISTANCE-SPECIFIC PLANS** including 100 Miler, with more coming soon.

3. **ROAD RUNNING PLANS** including Marathon 42.2 km, with more coming soon.

I love receiving feedback. Please take a moment to visit my website at **hannyallston.com.au** and send me some feedback.

Or perhaps you would like to come on one of my Trail Running Tours? Visit **findyourfeettours.com.au** to see what's coming up.

I love helping athletes. I would love to help you and to maybe run wilder on the trails with you, too.

Hanny Allston

About Hanny Allston

Hanny Allston is a familiar face in the Australian running scene. She is still the only non-European to win a World Orienteering Championship (2006), becoming the first athlete to win both the Junior and Senior titles in the same year. She 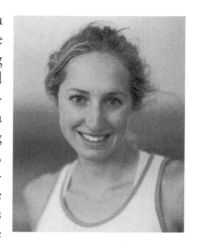 then progressed into marathon and distance track running, winning the Melbourne Marathon in 2007 and the New Zealand Marathon Championships in 2008. More recently she has enjoyed ultra- and trail-running successes, with two top-ten finishes on the World Skyrunning Series. She is the record holder for multiple trail- and ultra-running events across Australia. Today, her love affair lies in personal Missions, such as her 2017 12-hour traverse of Tasmania's South-Coast Track (GPS recorded distance 93 km) and 2018 11-hour summit of Federation Peak in Tasmania's remote South West Wilderness.

Hanny has always paired her athleticism with her non-sporting career. After studies in medical science, education, and life coaching, she founded Find Your Feet (established 2009), an award-winning outdoor retail, trail-running tourism and performance coaching company based in Tasmania, Australia.

Motivated to change the way people relate to themselves and the outdoors, Hanny pairs her business skills with an elite sporting background to create a powerful professional niche for herself. In 2015 she was awarded the Tasmanian Young Businesswoman of the Year and in 2018 her company was recognised as the Small & Succeeding Business in Tasmania.

Hanny's personal philosophy, stemming strongly from her life experiences, is 'Be Wilder. Play Wilder. Perform Wilder.'

For more information on Hanny please visit **hannyallston.com.au.**

About Find Your Feet

Founded by Hanny Allston, Find Your Feet strives to help you to Be, Play and Perform Wilder… to help you find your feet.

Their mission is to change the way we relate to ourselves and the outdoors by providing the highest quality athlete education, performance consulting, trail running tours and retail experiences. In 2018 the company was awarded the Small & Succeeding Business of the Year in Tasmania.

How Find Your Feet can help you:

- comprehensive online retail store, for all things trail running and adventurous!

- customised training planners for both marathon and trail running, including plans for specific events, trails and distances

- retail outlet in the heart of Australia's adventure capital, Hobart – located at 107 Elizabeth Street, Hobart, Tasmania

- educational and consulting services for people just like you!

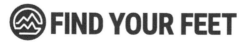

For more information please visit:

findyourfeet.com.au

Find Your Feet Trail Running Tours

Established in 2014, Find Your Feet's Trail Running Tours lead guests to exotic trail-running destinations, such as their home state of Tasmania in Australia, and further afield to the French Alps, Pyrenees, Italian Dolomites, Albania and Japan... just to name a few.

Find out more at:

findyourfeettours.com.au

.